SFIMMS SERIES IN NEUROMUSCULOSKELETAL MEDICINE

COUNTERSTRAIN APPROACHES
IN OSTEOPATHIC
MANIPULATIVE MEDICINE

Harry D. Friedman, D.O.
Wolfgang G. Gilliar, D.O.
Jerel H. Glassman, D.O.

Published by SFIMMS Press

San Francisco International Manual Medicine Society

email: admin@sfimms.com
www.sfimms.com

First Edition

Library of Congress Card Catalog Number 00-131504
ISBN 0-9701841-0-7

San Francisco International Manual Medicine Society

The San Francisco International Manual Medicine Society (SFIMMS) is an association of physicians and health professionals founded in 1995 to establish high educational standards and practice in the field of manual medicine.

The Society's courses are designed to provide health professionals with a strong foundation in manual medicine. The courses are offered at basic, intermediate and advanced levels with appropriate textbooks and course manuals provided. The educational format utilizes a variety of approaches including: Didactic Teaching, Step-By-Step Presentation, Hands-on Laboratory Sessions and Clinical Problem Solving.

These high quality educational programs facilitate the acquisition of palpatory skills and clinical problem solving approaches using a low student-teacher ratio in a direct, hands-on format.

Founding Members

Wolfgang G. Gilliar, DO (right)
Dr. Gilliar is in private practice in San Mateo, CA. He is board certified in Physical Medicine and Rehabilitation, and Osteopathic Manipulative Medicine. He is an assistant clinical professor at Michigan State University College of Osteopathic Medicine. He is also the editor and co-author of many Manual Medicine texts and scientific papers. Dr. Gilliar lectures and teaches extensively at national and international meetings. His specific research interests include neurophysiologic processes in their application to manual medicine and exercise principles, as well as practice parameter development.

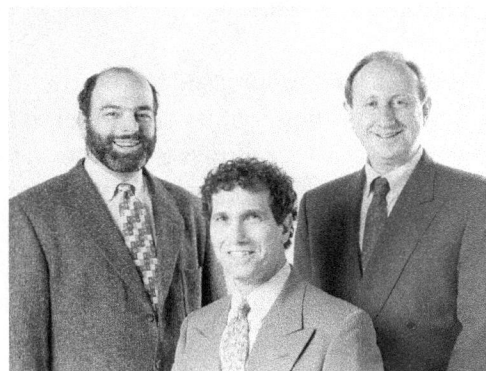

Harry D. Friedman, DO (left)
Dr Friedman is in private practice in Corte Madera, CA. He is board certified in Family Practice and Osteopathic Manipulative Medicine. He is an assistant clinical professor at Michigan State University College of Osteopathic Medicine and clinical faculty at Touro University College of Osteopathic Medicine.

Dr. Friedman has participated in various research studies concerning uniform osteopathic documentation. He is the author of a chapter for the Foundations of Osteopathic Medicine textbook and has co-authored the text Functional Methods. Dr. Friedman lectures and teaches extensively in the US and abroad, and is one of the faculty developing manual medicine programs for the American Academy of Family Physicians.

Jerel H. Glassman, MPH, DO (middle)
Dr. Glassman is a staff physician at St. Mary's Spine Center in San Francisco, CA. He is board certified in Physical Medicine and Rehabilitation, and Osteopathic Manipulative Medicine, and is an assistant clinical professor at Michigan State University College of Osteopathic Medicine and clinical faculty at Touro University College of Osteopathic Medicine. He is also a clinical instructor at Stanford University Medical School.

Dr. Glassman lectures frequently at many national meetings, including the American Academy of Physical Medicine and Rehabilitation, the American Back Society, the California Medical Association and American Osteopathic Association among others. Through his clinical and teaching activities he has pursued the integration of manual medicine into the multi-disciplinary rehabilitation model.

Foreward

The inspiration for this and the other books in the SFIMMS series in Neuromusculoskeletal Medicine came from our students and their desire for educational excellence. Quality instruction requires a level of clarity and correctness that reflects the subject's complexity but also allows for its comprehension on many different levels; conceptual, perceptual, and practical.

This material and the format in which it is presented have been developed to facilitate an understanding of Osteopathic Manipulative Medicine that encompasses its philosophy, science, and its practical clinical application. It is not the author's intention in writing this book to impart an Osteopathic education. Rather, we realize that such learning requires extensive study, supervision and clinical experience and cannot be acquired by simply reading this, or any other, book. We caution against the non-professional use of this book as it is intended as a textbook for Neuromusculoskeletal instruction in conjunction with a scientific education in the healing arts. Independent self-study of these approaches without the proper background and supervision is expressly against the authors' recommendation and wishes.

We were first impressed by the effectiveness of Dr. Jone's system. It's simple beauty combined with the boundless energy of its developer made it an approach we were immediately drawn to. As with all Osteopathic techniques the solution to the patients problem is made with a precise diagnosis. Dr. Jones' system offers just such great precision.

We wish to thank our teachers, Drs Lawrence Jones, DO, FAAO and Harold Schwartz, DO, FAAO for their inspiration and instruction. Our mentors at Michigan State University College of Osteopathic Medicine, and all the many colleagues and teachers who have helped us develop our Osteopathic approach. We want to especially thank our wives Denise, Barbara, and Beth for supporting us in our teaching and writing. And Eric Shilland for his many hours of computer support.

Contents

A Note on the Layout and Nomenclature of the Counterstrain Manual

This manual has been designed to serve as both a teaching text and a quick reference guide to counterstrain treatments. The general layout of the manual includes four parts for each treatment: a diagram indicating the location of the tender point, a photograph illustrating treatment position, an in-depth description of the tender point and treatment, and a graph to show at a glance which treatment positions will provide the greatest ease to the tender point. A sample treatment is shown below:

Treatment Description

Tender Point Location Diagram

Posterior Acromioclavicular (PAC)

Tender Pt. Posterior surface of lateral, superior acromion.

Treatment Patient prone. Operator places traction on arm from wrist.
Extension- slight
Adduction- slight
Traction- marked

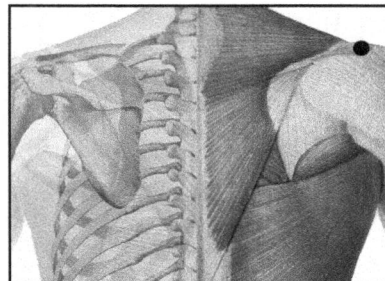

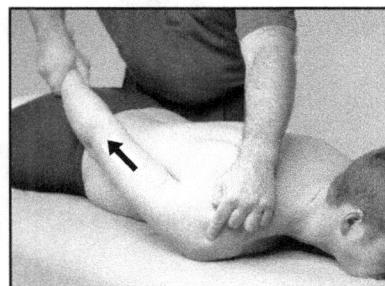

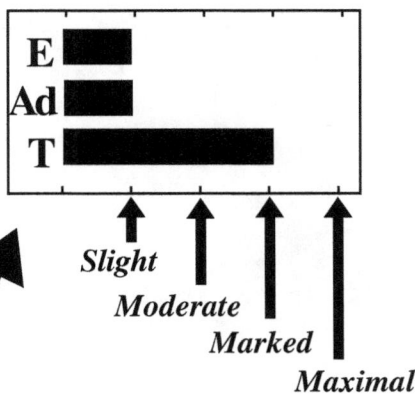

Treatment Graph

Slight

Moderate

Marked

Maximal

Treatment Position

The treatment graphs are meant to provide a quick reference for which positions will generally provide the most relief for tender points during treatment. Fine tuning of these movements should be done on a patient-by-patient basis. Each bar indicates a movement component of the treatment with the length indicating the relative amount of force needed. The following abbreviations are used in these graphs:

E = Extension	St = Sidebending towards point
F = Flexion	Sa = Sidebending away from point
C= Compression	In = Inversion
T = Traction	Ev = Eversion
Ri = Internal Rotation	Su = Supination
Re = External Rotation	Pr = Pronation
Ra = Rotation away from point	Ab = Abduction
Rt = Rotation towards point	Ad = Adduction

All of the tender points shown in this manual are demonstrated on the **right side** of the patient.

Introduction to Counterstrain

History of Counterstrain

Historically, osteopathic medicine has a long tradition of focusing on the malposition of one bone on another. Techniques to overcome this joint restriction have applied predominantly "direct" forces to put the joint back in its proper place. This conceptual framework has grown from the idea of a joint restriction or "blockage." Pain and its associated limited motions are the result of a restriction within the articular mechanism. Joint function is disturbed by repeated encounters with this restriction, and abnormal wear and tear on the articular components, including discs, may ensue. Treatment approaches have centered around breaking down this articular restriction, and so the familiar terminology "popping" the joints and "crunch" or "thrust" techniques have arisen.

Indirect methods have enjoyed a less illustrious, though surprisingly longer, history. Conceptually, these techniques defied explanation by bony positional relations and articular joint restrictions. In an early osteopathic text used at Kirksville College of Osteopathic Medicine, in 1915, indirect technique was described as the older of the two approaches. The indirect techniques were described as a traction method to relax the tissues about an articulation by exaggerating the forces or movements that produced the lesion. Lippincott described a similar approach in 1949 when reporting on the technique of William G. Sutherland:

> "The articulation is carried in the direction of the lesion, exaggerating the lesion position as far as necessary to cause the tension of the weakened elements of the ligamentous structure to be equal to or slightly in excess of the tension of those that were not strained. This is the point of balanced tension. When the tension is properly balanced, the respiratory or muscular cooperation of the patient is employed to overcome the resistance of the defense mechanism of the body to the release of the lesion."

The terminology for this type of procedure became known as a "balance-and-hold" technique.

Descriptions of indirect techniques challenged the mainstream conceptual framework of a joint restriction by focusing on the characteristics of the soft tissues surrounding the joint. Hoover and Bowles, credited with the development of functional indirect techniques, characterized the soft tissues not by their restrictions, but by their responses to paired motions as one of either ease or bind (i.e., one direction responds with decreasing tension – ease, the opposite direction with increasing tension - bind). This response information guides the technique in the direction of increasing soft tissue relaxation or ease.

The indirect concept recognizes a larger mobile system in which the joint and its surrounding tissues are a part, i.e., the motor system. Motor function, then, is a unique set of behaviors organized in response to demands placed on the entire system. Within that system are segmental reflexes that greatly influence the workings of the whole system.

Counterstrain Theory

Lawrence Jones, DO, in the early 1960's, developed an indirect method that he called spontaneous release by positioning, later renamed strain-counterstrain. He asserted that tissue tension about a strained joint did not splint in order to prevent movement into the strain position, but to resist movement away from the strain position. He taught that even the most severe strains would tolerate being returned to the position in which the strain originally occurred, and only to this position.

Jones made his "discovery" quite by accident while trying to offer symptomatic relief to a patient experiencing treatment failure. After suffering four months from a low back condition that prevented the patient from standing erect, Jones tried to help him find a comfortable position in which to sleep. Propping the patient with pillows, Jones helped the man find a pain-free position with maximal hip flexion. After 20 minutes, the patient was still pain-free and when Jones assisted him off the table, he was able to stand up straight for the first time in four months. Jones was so surprised at the quick resolution of this stubborn case that he was determined to understand what had happened.

Jones experimented with positions of comfort and noticed frequent treatment success. He was able to find and relieve tender spots in the muscles that were in spasm; however, some patients would return with the same problem he had treated previously. After successfully treating a groin injury by locating a tender spot in the anterior pelvis, Jones began to search the anterior side of patients with these chronic persistent paravertebral spasms. His search was again met with success as he often found spasm and tender spots in the antagonist muscles to those in pain. As Jones developed these ideas he brilliantly linked together the relationship of joint mechanics with muscle attachments. He refined the osteopathic approach to segmental somatic dysfunction by considering it's anterior and posterior relationships.

When a strain occurs, tissues about a joint are stretched (*e.g.* Muscle A) while antagonist tissues are shortened (*e.g.* Muscle B). When stretched, Muscle A increases its proprioceptive feedback to protect it from overstretching. Muscle B, its antagonist, needs little protective proprioceptive feedback in its shortened state. (See Figures 1 & 2). Muscle A reacts to being suddenly stretched by reflexly contracting, presumably a protective response. Muscle B will then be suddenly stretched by Muscle A's reflex contraction. (See Figure 3). In a state of relative proprioceptive silence, Muscle B's sudden stretch will signal a strong rise in proprioceptive feedback, registering a stretch of that muscle even though no stretch has actually occurred. (Muscle B is actually at about its normal resting length.) Muscle B reacts to this sudden change in proprioceptive output like it would to an actual stretch: it reflexly contracts. (See Figure 4). Because of the sudden increase in Muscle B's spindle activity, what was previously its resting length and resting tone now assumes a hypertonic tone in a contracted state. Muscle A recovers from its reflex contraction and strain, but becomes inhibited and painful due to the unresolved counterstrain in Muscle B. Muscle B's sustained hypertonus is then thought to lead to myofascial and neurovascular disturbances described clinically as a "tender point".

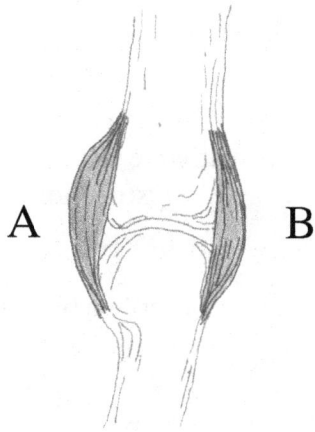

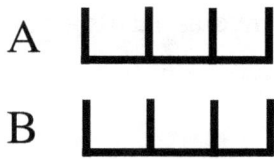

Figure 1: Normal Resting Tone

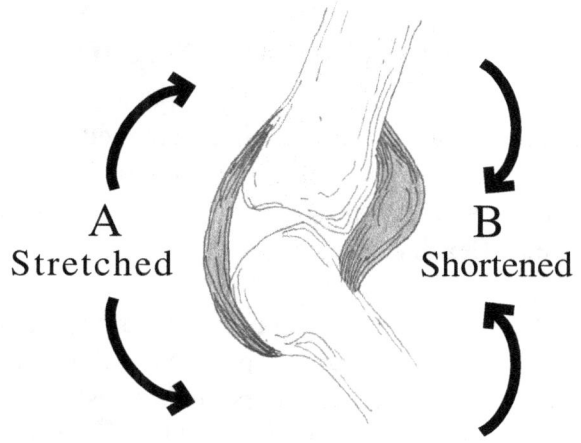

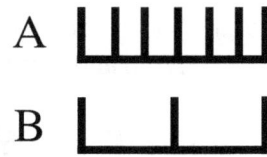

Figure 2: Strain

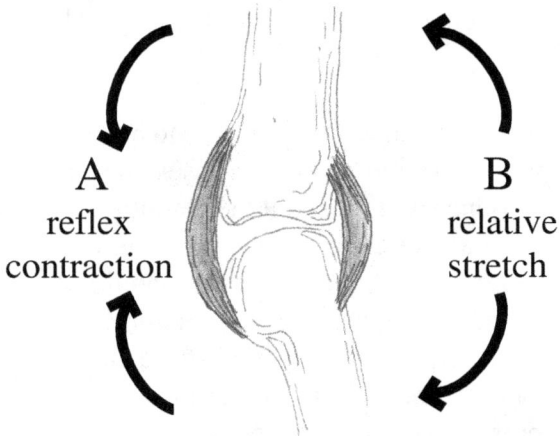

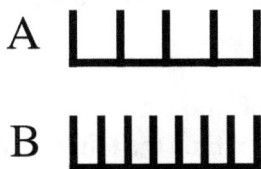

Figure 3: Counterstrain

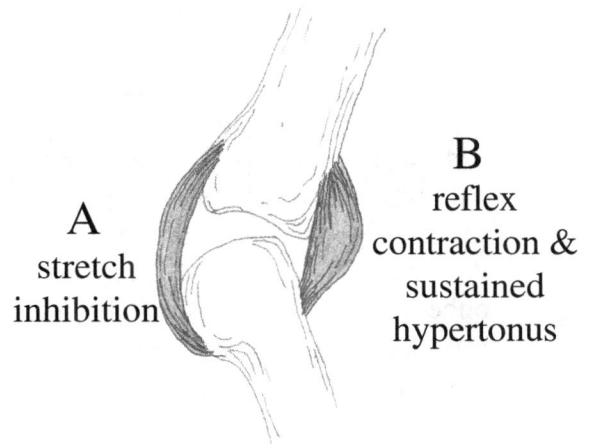

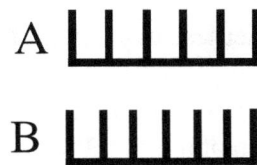

Figure 4: Dysfunctional Resting Tone

Definition of Counterstrain

Counterstrain is an indirect manipulative medicine technique in which tenderness (of a tender point) is relieved by patient positioning to a point of comfort or ease away from the restrictive barrier. A position of mild but asymptomatic strain is reproduced, which over time releases somatic dysfunction and its associated reflex disturbances.

The counterstrain tender point is not the same as a myofascial trigger point, as described by Travell and Simon. The myofascial trigger point has a characteristic pain pattern that radiates away from the trigger point. The counterstrain tender point demonstrates local tenderness only. Tender points additionally correspond to somatic dysfunctions of the associated spinal or appendicular joint or soft tissue complex, where the actual strain has thought to have occurred. Myofascial trigger points have a local pathology independent of the surrounding joints and soft tissues. Treatment approaches also differ; in counterstrain the somatic dysfunction is treated by shortening hypertonic muscles, while myofascial trigger points often require injections, stretch and spray or other techniques.

Counterstrain Treatment Method

1. **Finding the tender point**. Tender points are associated with areas of somatic dysfunction, as mentioned earlier. By performing a musculoskeletal screening examination, general problem areas can be identified and related tender points located. Often, the patient's history explaining the mechanism of injury will shed light on the location of dysfunctional forces impacting the body. The patient may be splinting in a particular way that indicates the direction of forces and the position of injury that the patient is protecting.

    Using the finger pads to locate the tender points is superior to using the tips of the fingers. These points are tense, often swollen, and occasionally nodular, eliciting tenderness with just slight pressure into the center of the point.

2. **Establish baseline tenderness assessment.** Tenderness is a subjective response to nociceptor stimulation, the perception of which can vary from patient to patient. In most cases, the tender point will be quite sensitive to pressure; however, experience will often tell the practitioner that the tender point is clinically relevant, even if the patient has a relative lack of tenderness. In either case, the patient should be asked if the point is tender. Next, the tenderness should be graded as mild, moderate, or intense. Pushing on the tender point a few times is helpful to familiarize the patient with the most precise character of the pain elicited. Each time the tender point is palpated, the operator should hold pressure for only one to two seconds and then the pressure on the tender point is released. Never hold pressure on the tender point continuously. Whatever the intensity of the tenderness, have the patient assign this a $100 value as a baseline of tenderness in the point before treatment.

3. **Reduce the tenderness by placing the patient in a position of maximal comfort.** The position of maximal patient comfort is defined by the position in which the tender point is maximally reduced in its intensity. Ideally, this should be at least a 70% reduction in tenderness to be a therapeutic position of comfort. The position of maximal patient comfort is usually the

same as the patient's position at the time of the injury that caused the dysfunction. It is often helpful to start treatment with the patient in a position that simulates the position of injury. Check the tender point for reduction of pain and then fine tune to the position of maximal comfort. The greater the reduction of tenderness, the more effective is the treatment.

Maintain light contact over the tender point throughout the procedure in order to re-check the point tenderness, if necessary, and to re-check the same point after treatment. Additionally, changes in the tender point will be evident at various points in the treatment procedure. At the start, upon finding the position of maximal patient comfort, the tension in the tender point will ease up, and at the end of the treatment, when the somatic dysfunction releases, the tender point will pulsate. This pulsation signals the end of the treatment procedure, and usually occurs after about 90 seconds.

4. **Hold the position of maximal patient comfort for 90 seconds.** During this time, the patient (and operator) must be relaxed. Often patients need to be reminded several times to let go of tension that may creep back into the treated areas.

Each treatment can be carried out with different operator positions to accomplish the same position of comfort for the patient. Knowing multiple approaches to any given technique will help the operator to find an optimal position of comfort that fits the patient's situation.

5. **Slowly return the patient to a neutral position.** After the tender point has released (in approximately 90 seconds), return the patient to a neutral position without any patient effort whatsoever. The operator must instruct the patient to stay completely relaxed while the operator slowly brings the patient (passively) back to neutral. Any patient effort will negatively influence the benefit from the treatment. If the patient has a guarding reaction, the operator should stop the return movement and wait for the patient to relax before moving again.

6. **Re-test the tender point.** Once the patient is returned to a neutral resting position, the operator will re-test the tender point. The patient should compare the amount of tenderness to the original $100 of tenderness. Any more than $30 remaining is a poor response and should be re-treated. All aspects of the somatic dysfunction associated with the tender point should also show signs of improvement, including myofascial and ligamentous relaxation, spindle cell and motor control recalibration, vasodilation, and waste product wash-out. (See clinical correlations for additional information on counterstrain treatment methods.)

Summary of Counterstrain Treatment Method

1. Find the tender point.
2. Establish baseline tenderness assessment.
3. Reduce the tenderness by placing the patient in a position of maximal comfort.
4. Hold the position of maximal patient comfort for 90 seconds.
5. Slowly return the patient to a neutral position.
6. Re-test the tender point.

Clinical Considerations

The history of the patient often gives clues as to the location and type of tender point you are likely to find. Observing the patient's body position and posture may reflect focal points of stress (e.g. tender points) around which the body is bent, folded or otherwise engaged.

The treatment protocol for each tender point is only a starting point; fine tuning is always necessary to individualize the patient's response. In a small percentage of patients, treatment protocol will not reach a therapeutic reduction of the tender point. In these cases, the protocol should be reversed to attempt to achieve therapeutic results. Starting with rotation or side-bending, the opposite position is then introduced. If side-bending right is recommended in the protocols, then side-bending left should be used. If side-bending and rotation are not sufficient, change the direction between flexion and extension.

Another situation may also be interfering with the desired therapeutic response. The stubborn tender point may be a secondary response to a more primary tender point located elsewhere. Often, anterior and posterior points of the same segment have such primary-secondary relations. Locating and treating these related tender points may result in a more favorable therapeutic outcome.

Frequently, somatic dysfunctions associated with tender points will return when a patient resumes normal activities too soon, or if the similar strain should occur, as the patient is more vulnerable to a recurrence of the original.

To reduce spasm and help facilitate the patient's return to more optimal motor responses, home positioning can be incorporated between treatments. Once a significant tender point has been treated, the patients can be instructed to position themselves similarly at home with the use of pillows, couches, chairs, beds, etc. Assistance by a spouse or family member is often helpful to get the patient into and out of such positions of maximal comfort at home. Caution must be used when resuming the position of maximal comfort, as injury may occur from too great a patient effort. Home positioning should be reserved, then, for recurrences only.

Anterior Cervical Tender Points

Typically, the anterior cervical tender points are located on the antero-lateral aspect of the lateral masses. There are atypical locations for the first, seventh, and eighth anterior cervical tender points. Anterior tender points typically require flexion, rotation, and sidebending away from the tender point. AC7 may require sidebending towards the tender point. The AC3 tender point may require extension.

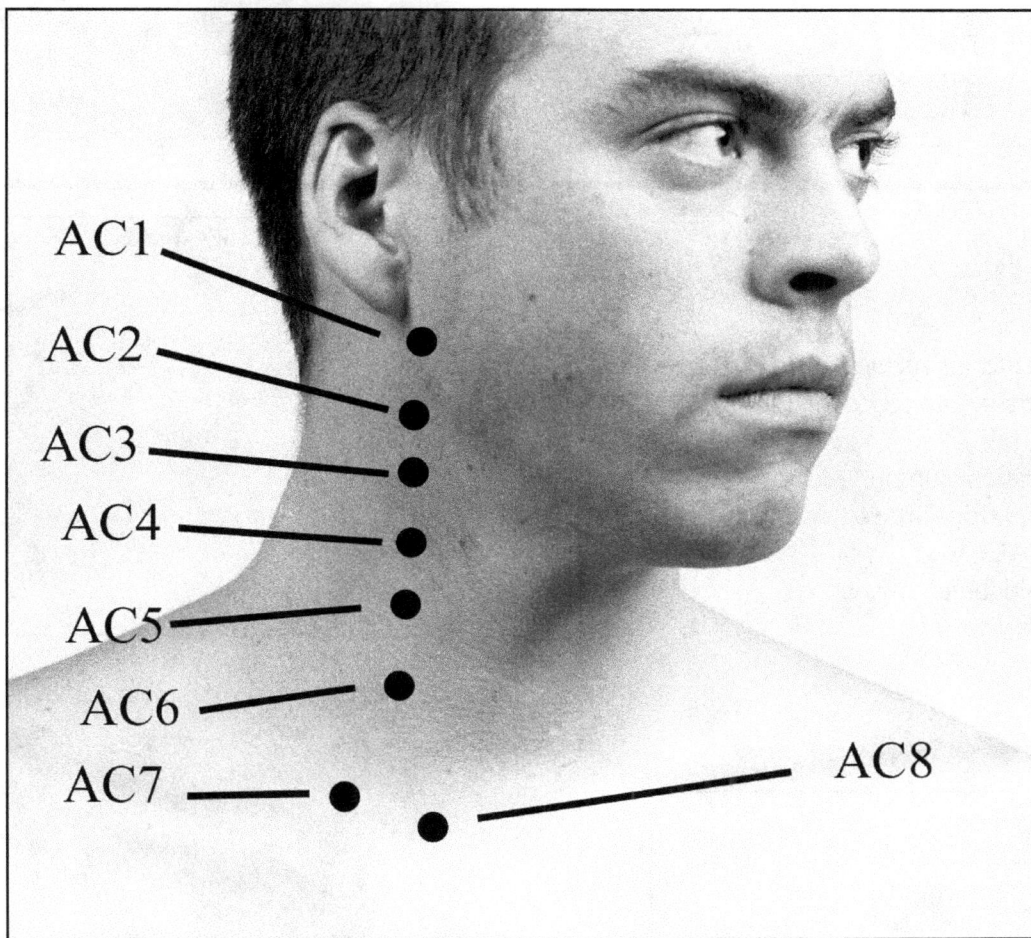

AC1

Tender Pt.   Posterior surface of ascending ramus of
mandible, superior to the angle.
Approach TP posteriorly.

Treatment   Patient supine.
Flexion or extension- little or none
Sidebend away slightly
Rotate away markedly. Patient's head
rests on operator's hand. Operator may
need to apply some pressure to the side of
the patient's head with their other hand,
adding more sidebending away (into the
table).

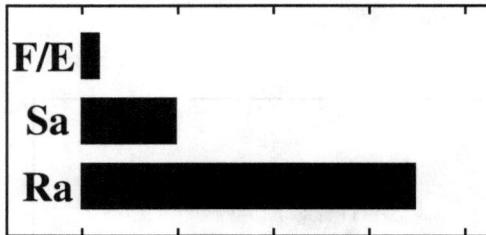

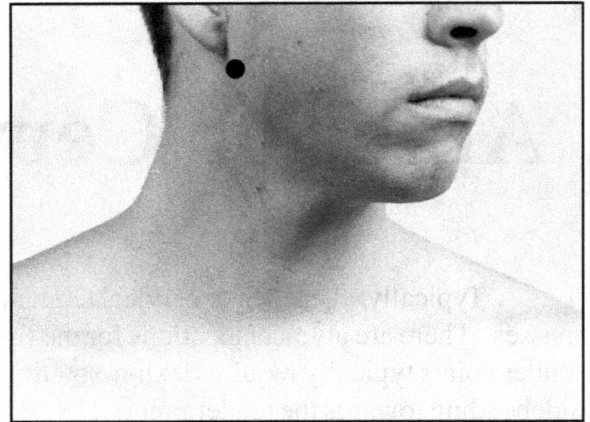

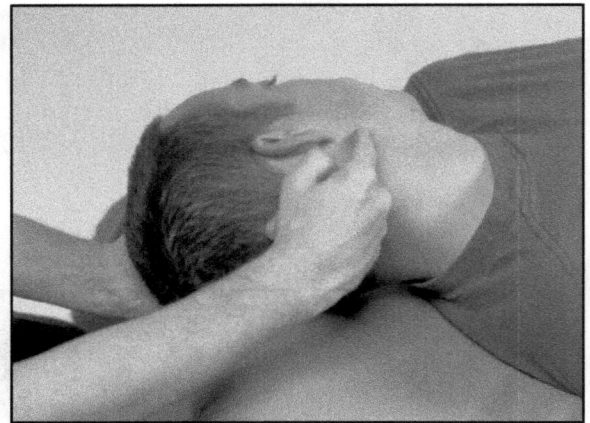

F/E	▮
Sa	▬▬▬
Ra	▬▬▬▬▬▬

AC 2,4-6

AC2
AC4
AC5
AC6

Tender Pt.   Anterior surface of tip of corresponding
transverse process.

Treatment   Patient supine.
Flexion- little to moderate (more for AC5 &
  AC6).
Sidebend- away.
Rotate- away.

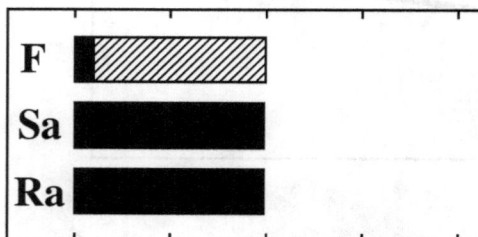

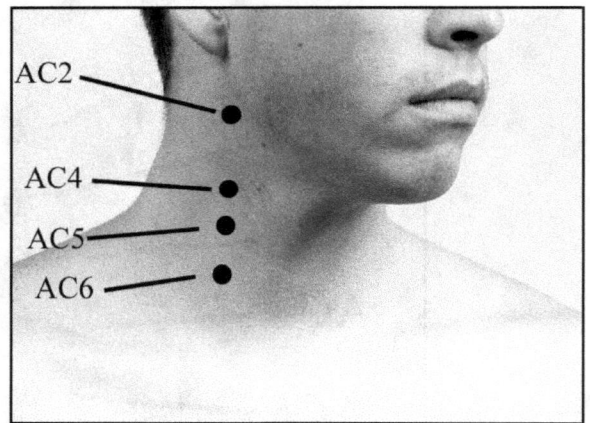

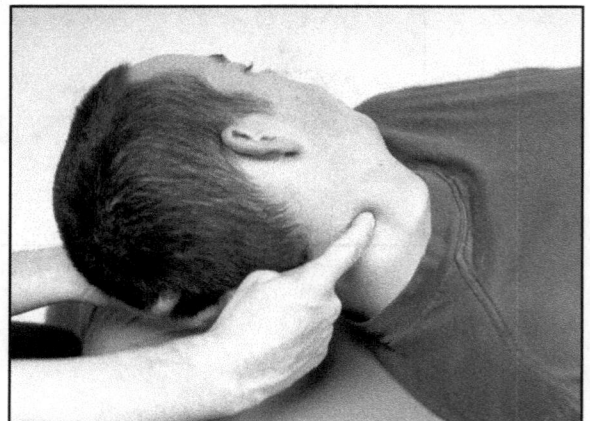

F	▨▨▨
Sa	▬▬▬
Ra	▬▬▬

AC3

Tender Pt.   Anterior surface of tip of C3 transverse process.

Treatment   Patient supine.
Extension- slight.
Sidebend- away.
Rotate- away.

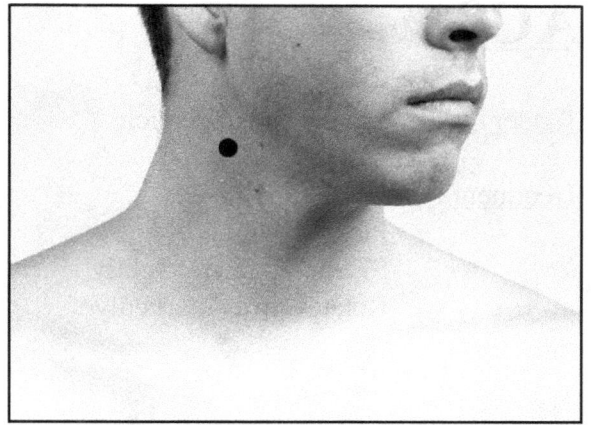

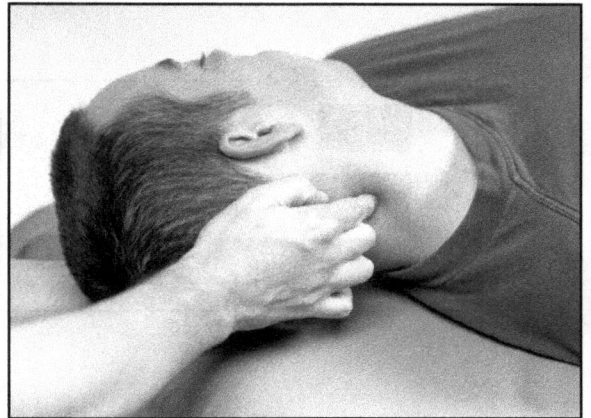

E	
Sa	
Ra	

AC7

Tender Pt.   About 2 cm lateral to medial end of clavicle on superior, posterior surface.

Treatment   Patient supine.
Flexion- marked, of low neck.
Sidebend- toward markedly.
Rotate- away slightly.

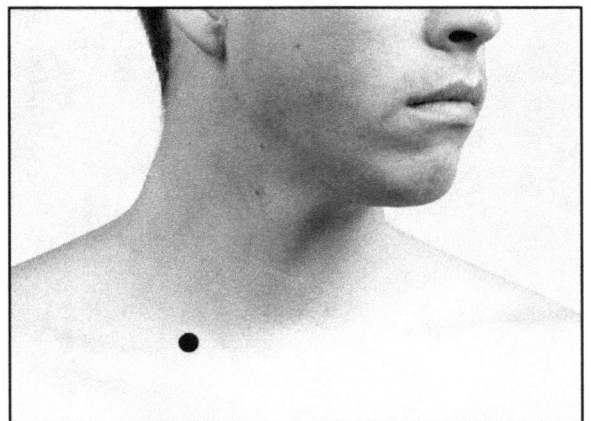

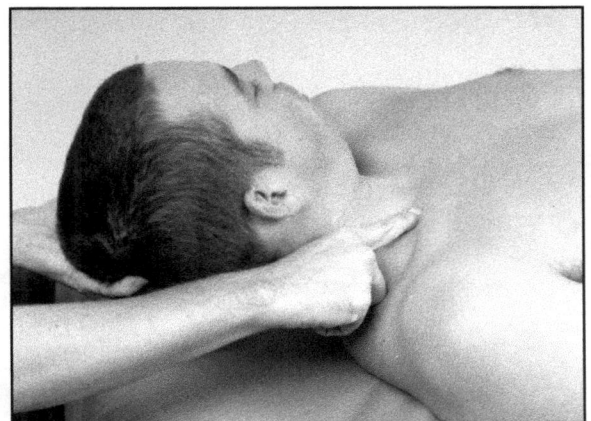

F	
St	
Ra	

AC8

Tender Pt.   Medial end of clavicle.

Treatment   Patient supine.
Flexion- slight.
Sidebend- away slightly.
Rotate- away markedly.

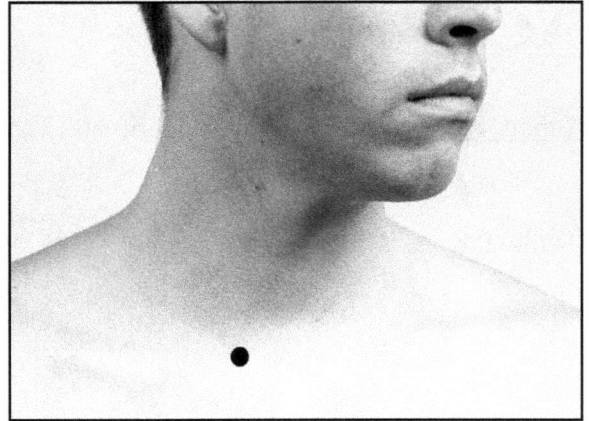

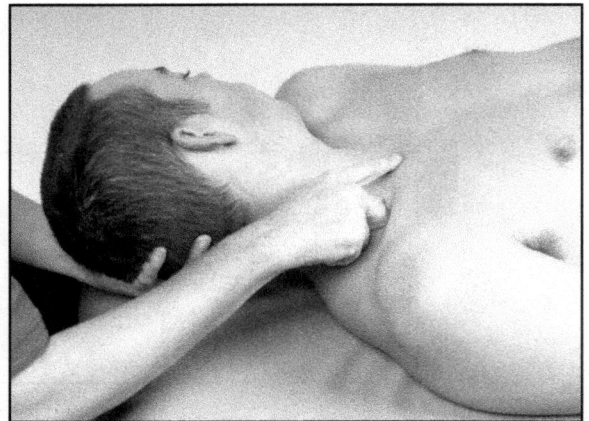

F	
Sa	
Ra	

Posterior Cervical Tender Points

The posterior cervical tender points are generally associated with the lateral aspects of the tips of the spinous processes. Sometimes tender points will be found in the paraspinal myofascial tissue just lateral to the spinous processes. Atypical tender points are found at the top and bottom of the posterior cervical spine with the first, second, and eighth posterior points located in atypical places. Posterior cervical tender points typically require extension, rotation, and sidebending away from the tender point. The PC1 inion requires marked flexion.

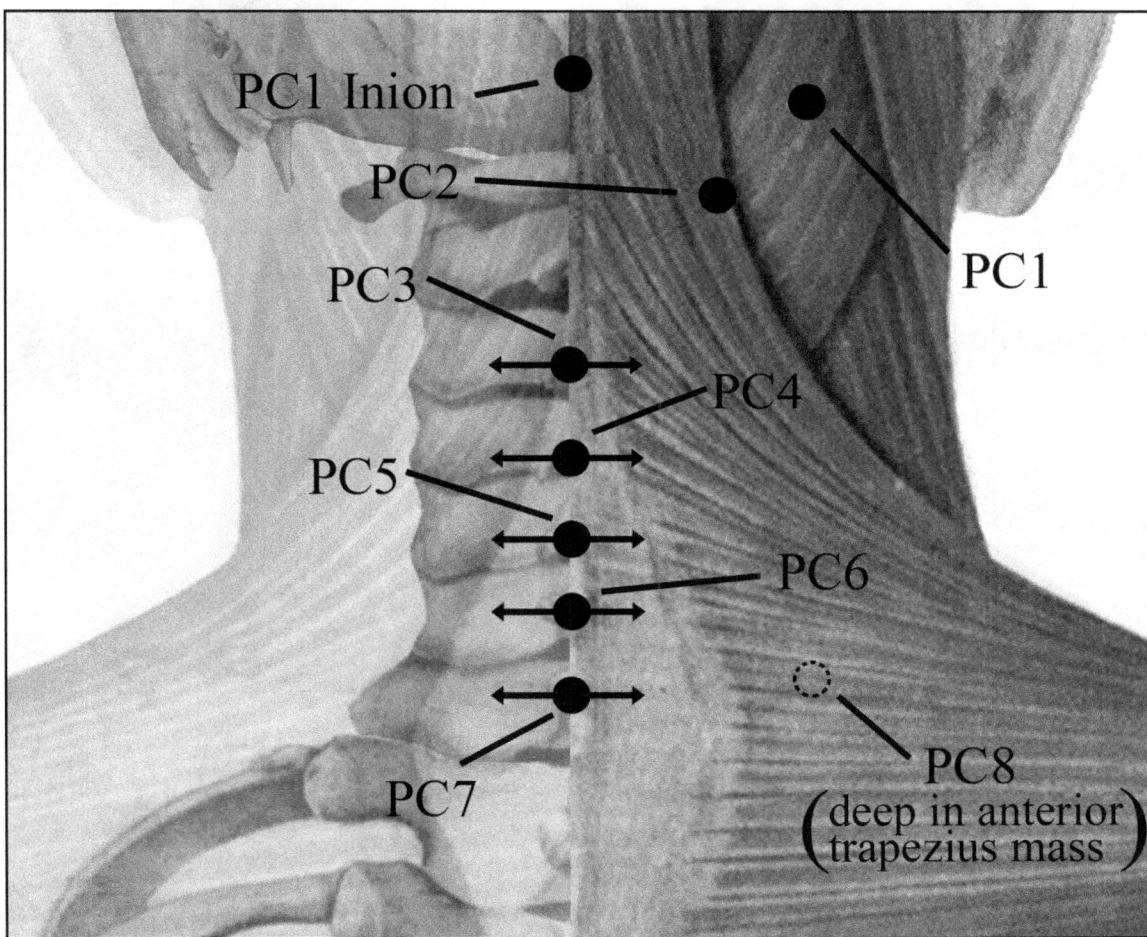

PC1-2

Tender Pt.
PC1- On occiput lateral to main muscle mass. 3-4 cm from midline.

PC2- On lateral border of main muscle mass of neck just below occiput. 2 cm lateral to midline.

Treatment
Patient supine.
Extension- at level of C1/C2. Lift head to flex lower cervicals allowing marked extension of C1/C2.
Sidebend- away slightly.
Rotate- away some. Augment extension of C1/C2 by hand pressure on top of head

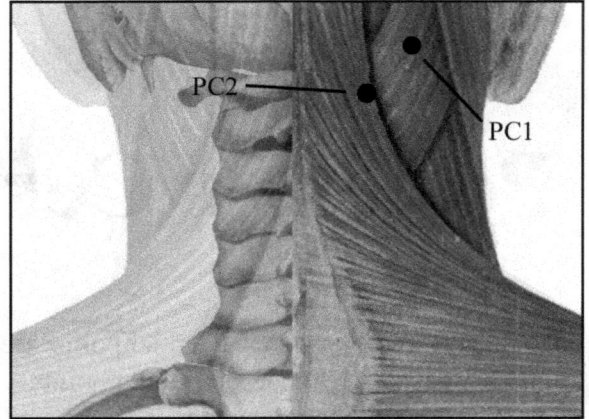

E	████████████
Sa	███
Ra	█████

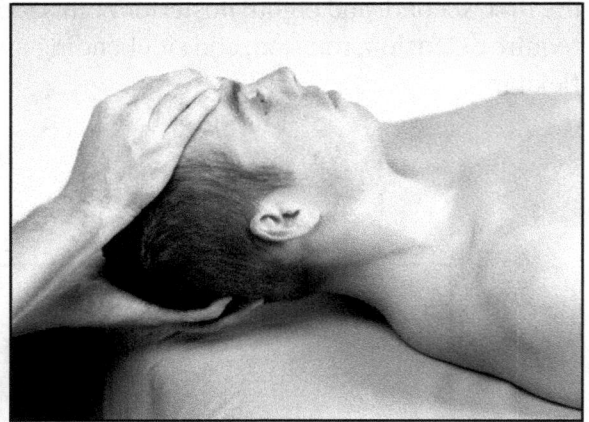

PC1 Inion

Tender Pt.
On medial border of main muscle mass of neck 2 cm below inion.

Treatment
Patient supine. Gentle but firm head control is very important.
Flexion- maximal.
Sidebend- toward slightly.
Rotate- away slightly.

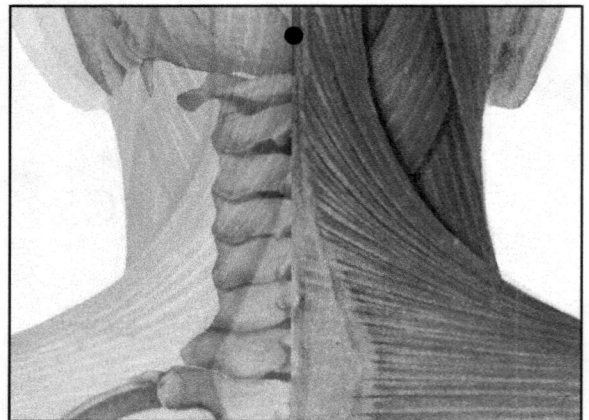

F	████████████
St	███
Ra	███

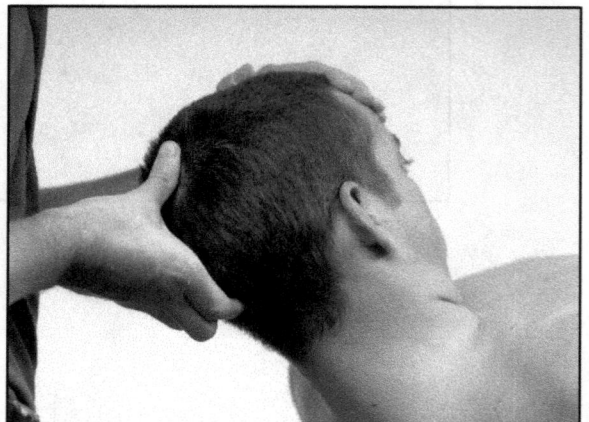

14

PC3-7

<u>Tender Pts.</u> On spinous process of corresponding cervical level or in muscle mass between spinous and transverse processes.

<u>Treatment</u> Patient supine with head extended over the end of table. The more the head is extended, the lower the action from PC4 through PT2.
Extension- moderate to marked, more for lower cervicals.
Sidebend- away.
Rotate- away.
PC3 tender points are rare, most C3 dysfunctions are treated anteriorly.

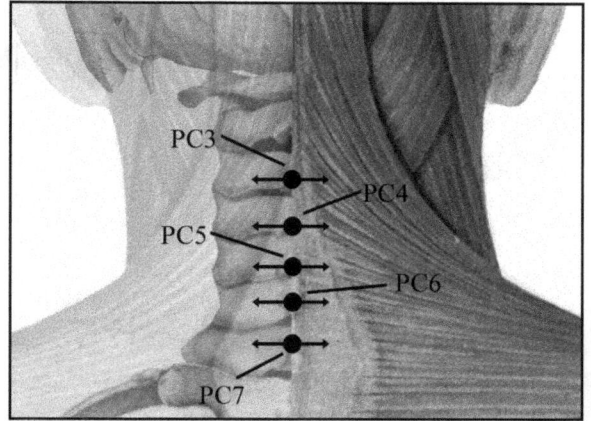

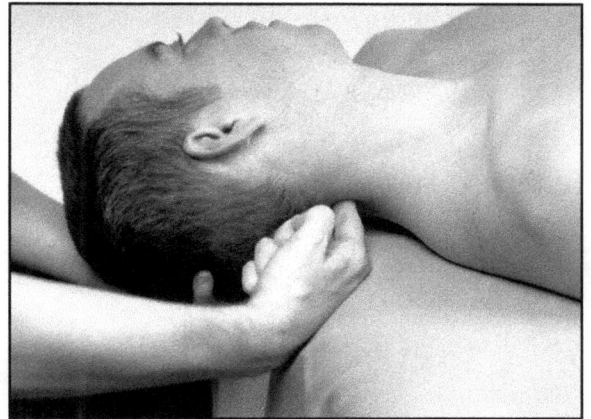

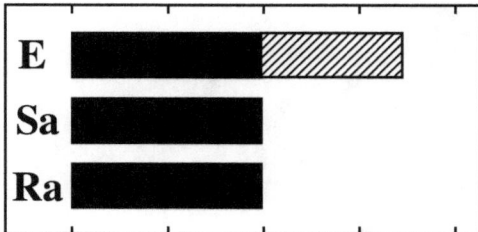

PC8

<u>Tender Pt.</u> Anterior to the trapezius mass at the base of the neck on the posterior surface of tip of transverse process of C7.

<u>Treatment</u> Patient supine or prone.
Extension- slight
Sidebend- away markedly
Rotate- away

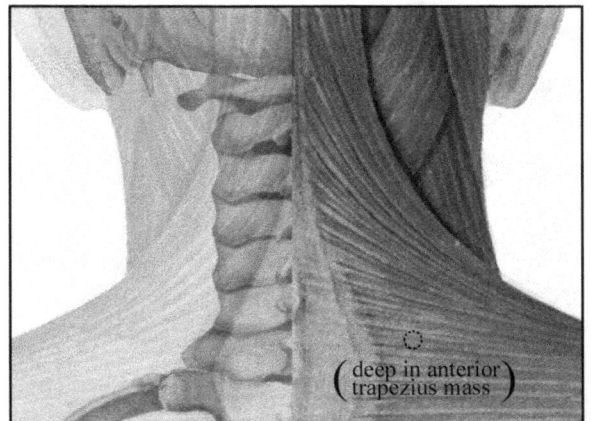

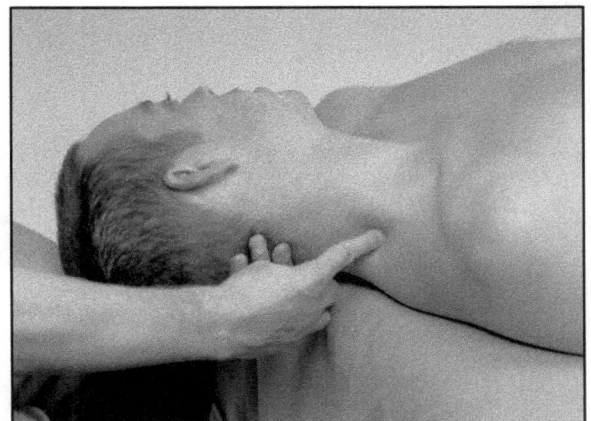

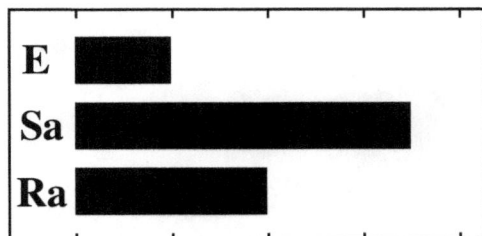

<u>Notes</u>

Anterior Thoracic Tender Points

The anterior thoracic spine tender points are located in two major areas. The first group of tender points, AT1-7, are located midline on the sternum. They can be located by palpating for tenderness and tissue tension overlying the sternum. The second group of tender points are located in the abdominal wall, most are located in the rectus abdominis muscle on the midline or laterally about one or two centimeters from the midline. These anterior tender points most often require flexion, rotation and sidebending away from the tender point. Tender points may also be located on the upper aspect of the inferior costal margin or in the interspaces of the false ribs. These tender points typically require some flexion, sidebending toward and rotation away from the tender point.

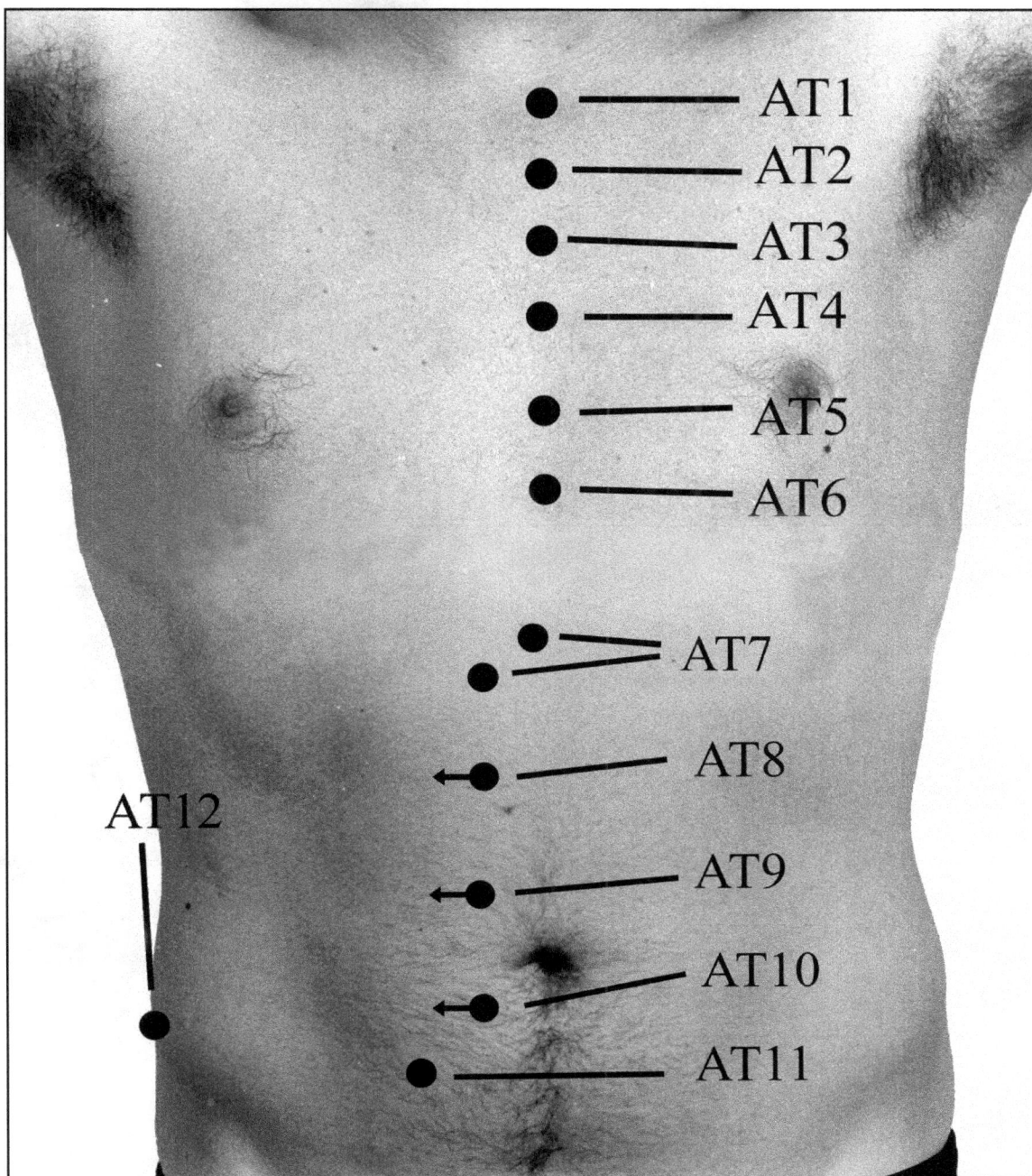

AT1
AT2
AT3
AT4
AT5
AT6
AT7
AT8
AT12
AT9
AT10
AT11

AT1-6

Tender Pts.   AT1- Midline in suprasternal notch.

AT2- Middle of manubrium in midline.

AT3- 2-2.5 cm below manubrium junction.

AT4- 5 cm below manubrium junction, at the level of 4th interspace.

AT5/6- Level of 5th and 6th interspaces on anterior midline of sternum

Treatment   Patient supine. Operator at head of table with knee on table. Operator flexes patient at level of tender point while supporting neck and spine with hand and thigh.
Flexion- marked

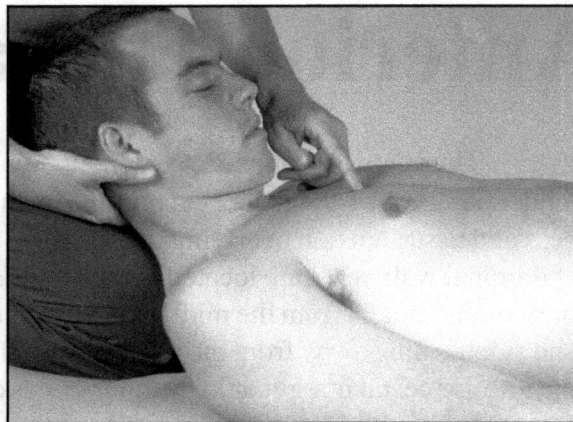

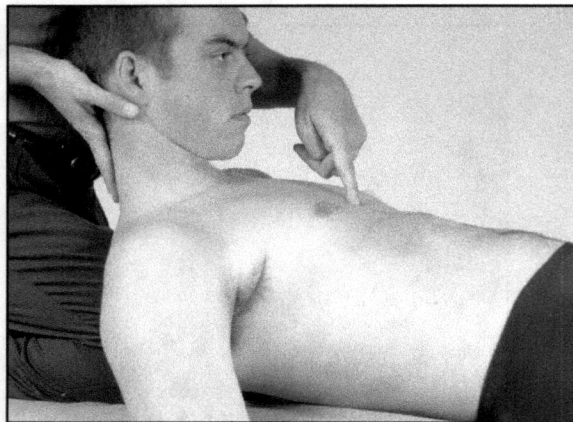

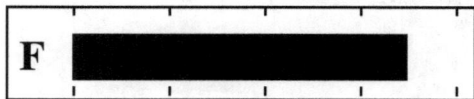

F ████████████

Alternate Treatment for AT1-6

Treatment   Patient seated with hands on top of head. Operator places arms around patient under axilla and locks hands over the manubrium/sternum inducing flexion to the tender point..
Flexion- marked

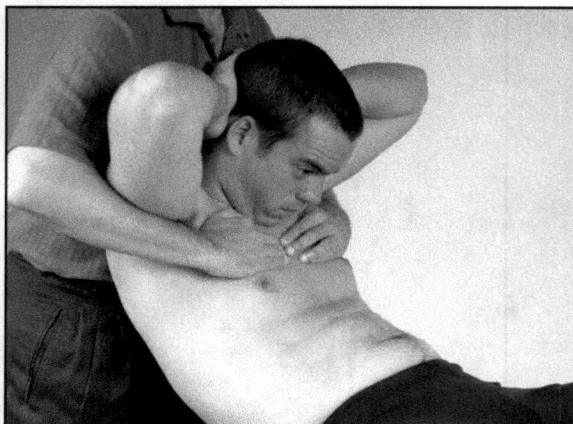

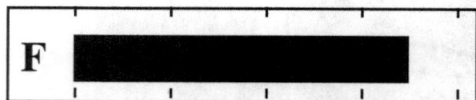

F ████████████

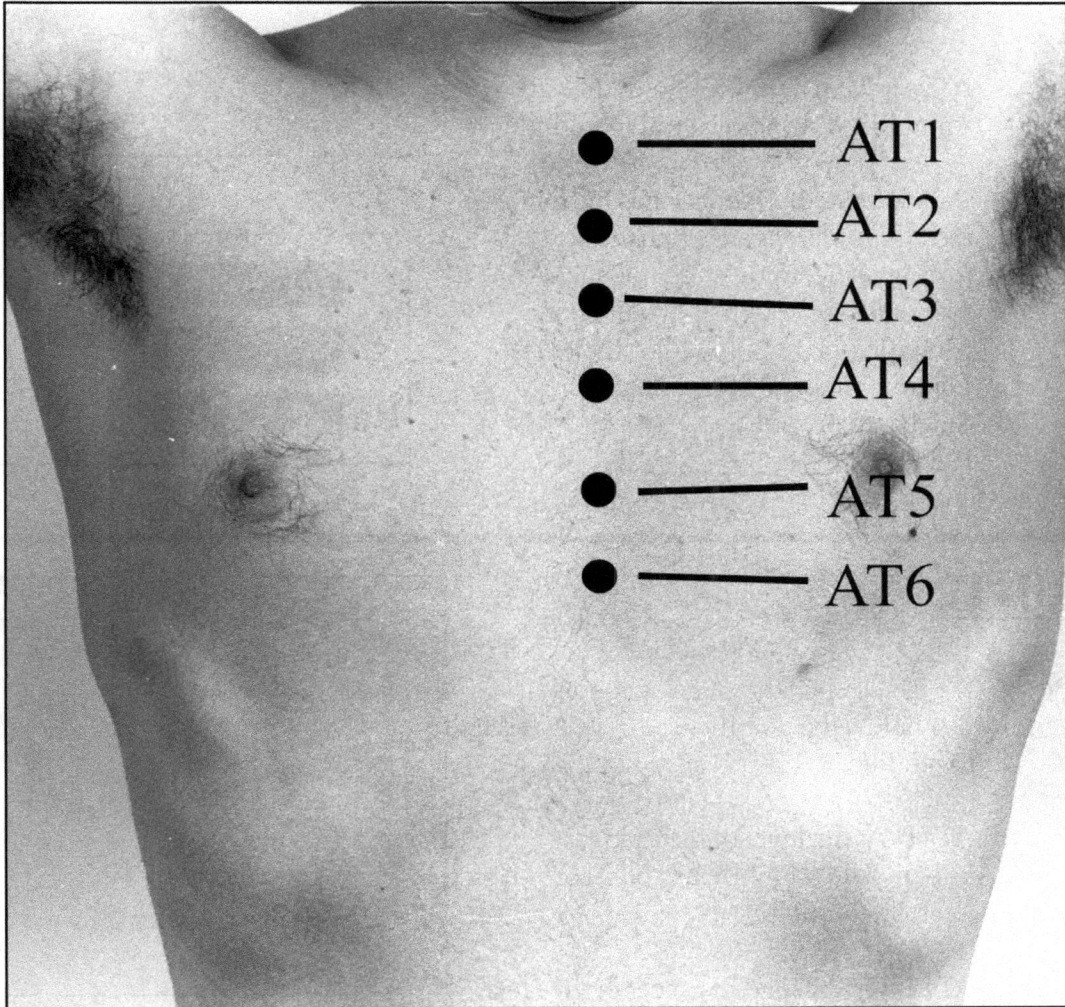

Tender Points for Anterior Thoracics 1-6

AT7-9

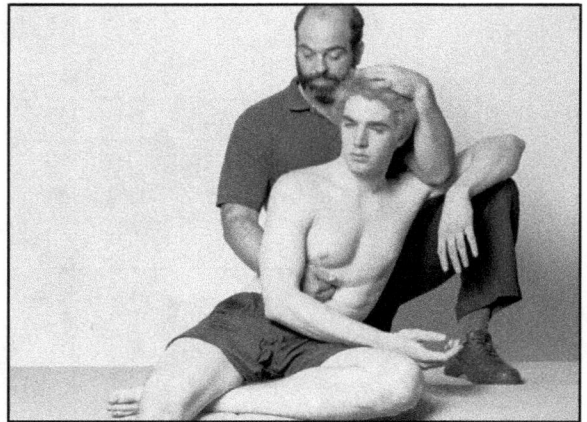

<u>Tender Pts.</u>   AT7- On or 1 cm below the xiphoid, 1 cm lateral to midline.

AT8- 3-4 cm below xiphoid, 2-3 cm lateral to midline.

AT9- 6-7 cm below xiphoid. Just above umbilicus, 1-3 cm lateral to midline.

<u>Treatment</u>   Patient seated. Operator has his foot on the table. Patient has opposite arm resting on operator's thigh. Patient's foot on table on side of dysfunction. More flexion required for AT8 & AT9.
Flexion- moderate to marked.
Sidebend- toward.
Rotate- away.

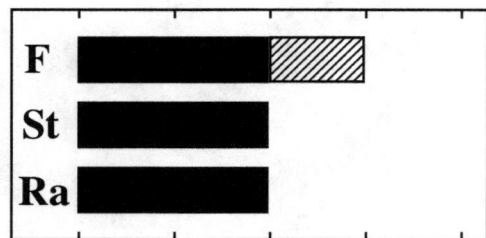

AT10-12

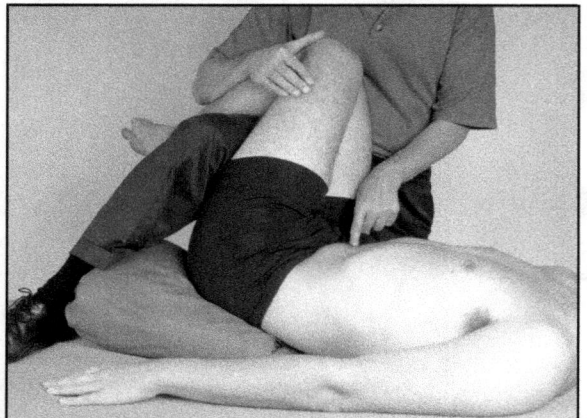

<u>Tender Pts.</u>   AT10- Deep in the anterior abdomen just below the umbilicus, 1-3 cm lateral to midline.

AT11- At the level of the iliac crest, 3-4 cm below umbilicus and 3 cm lateral to midline.

AT12- On the medial aspect of the crest of the ilium in the midaxillary line.

<u>Treatment</u>   Patient supine. Place several pillows under hips of the patient to obtain flexion of pelvis on lumbar spine. Operator stands on the side of the dysfunction with patient's flexed legs on thigh. Produce marked flexion at the level of the dysfunction. AT9 can also be treated supine if flexion is increased up to T9 level.
Flexion.
Sidebend- toward.
Rotate- away.(legs towards sore side induces relative rotation of torso away)

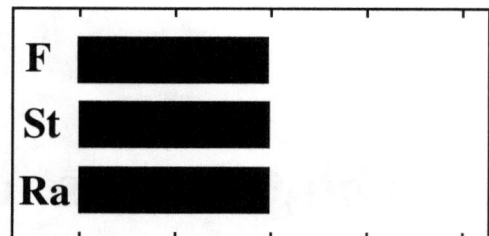

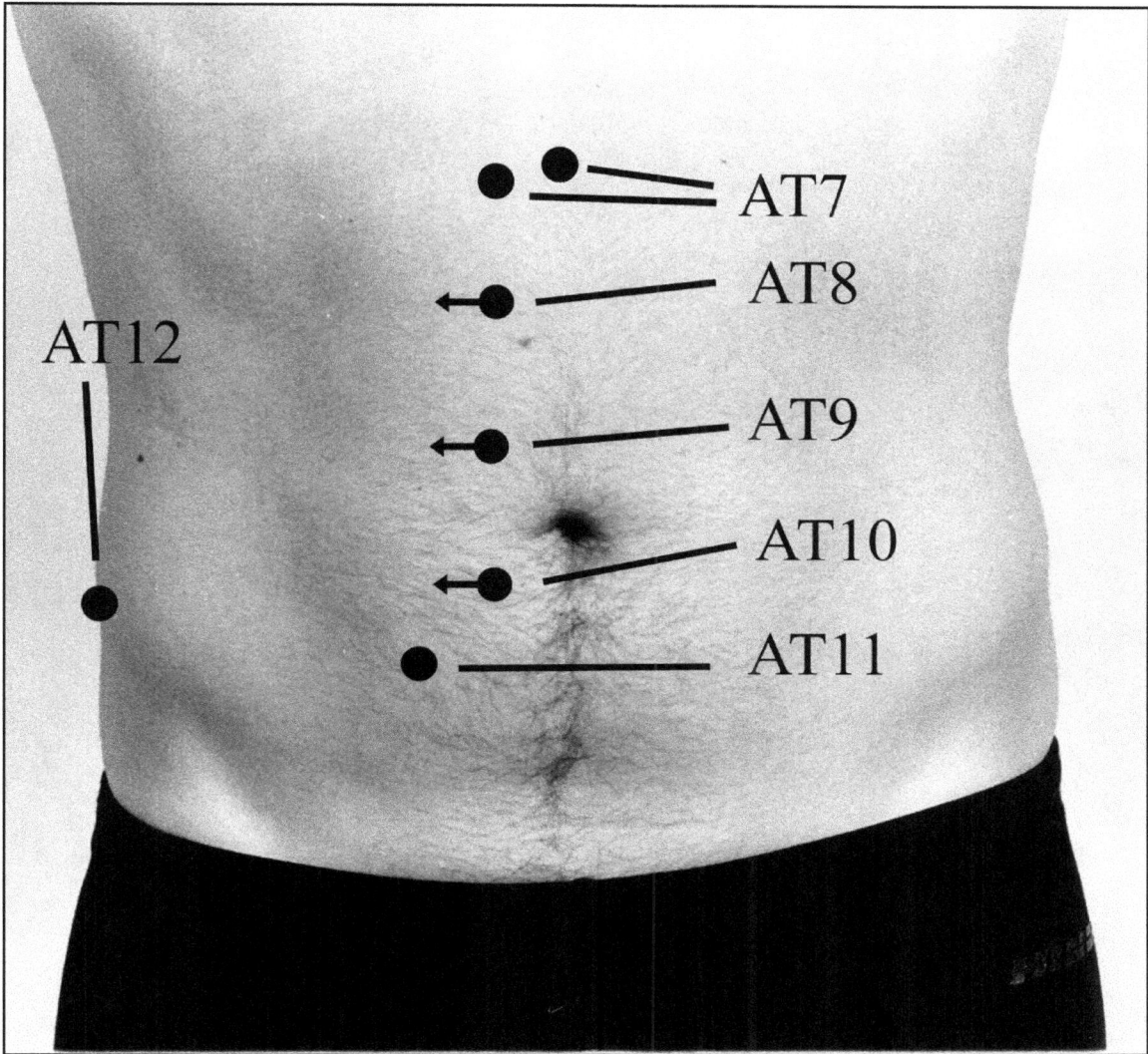

Tender Points for Anterior Thoracics 7-12

Notes

Posterior Thoracic Tender Points

The posterior thoracic tender points can be found in two locations on each vertebra. One location is associated with the tip of the spinous process (SP), often just lateral to the tip. The second location is on the tip of the transverse process (TP) on either side. The tender points on the spinous processes typically require extension. Those on the transverse processes are rountinely treated with extension, rotation towards, and sidebending away from the tender point. With posterior upper thoracic tender points, the closer the tender point is to the midline, the more force in extension is needed. The further the tender point is located from the midline, the more sidebending is needed.

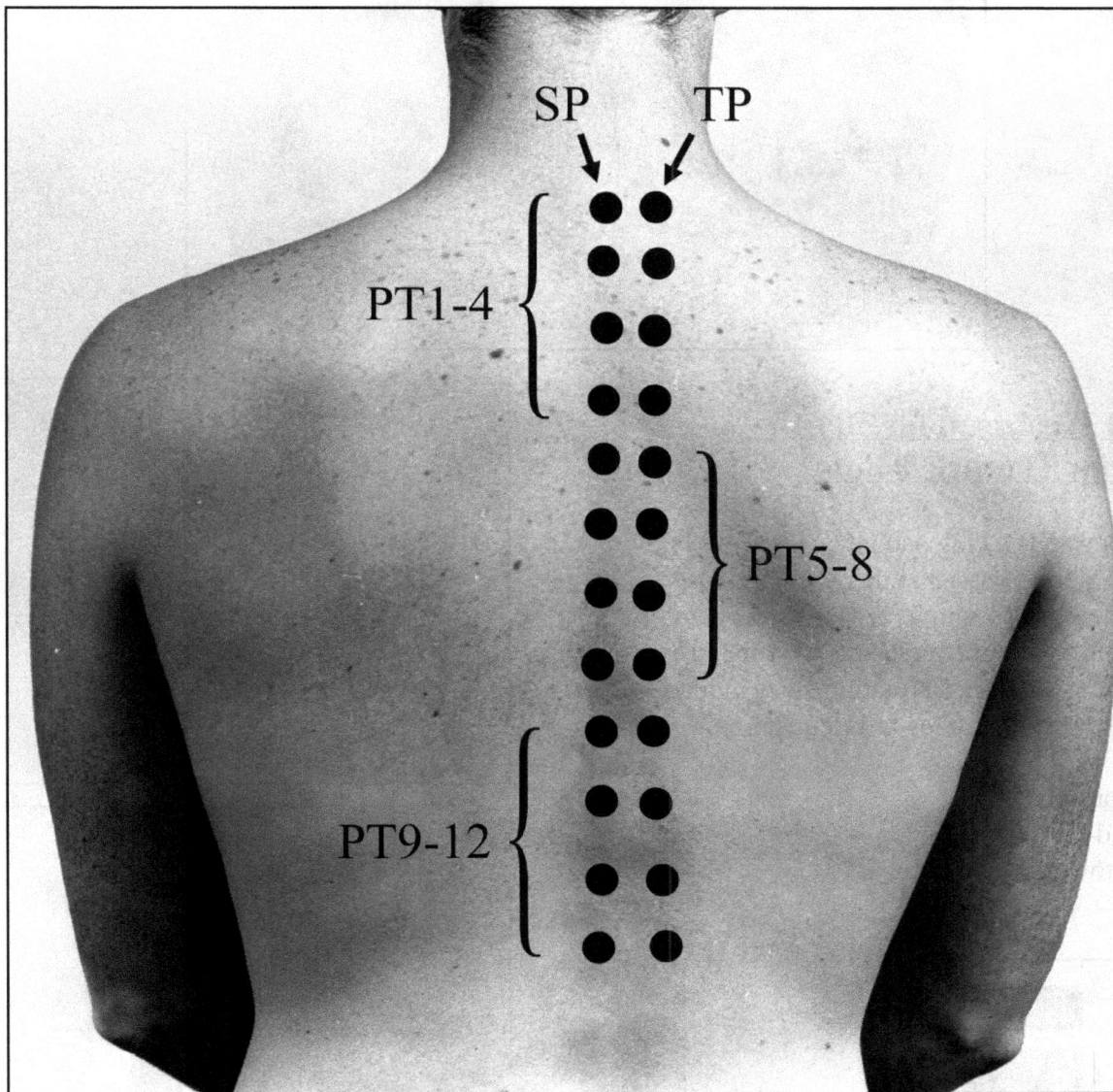

Posterior Thoracic Tender Points

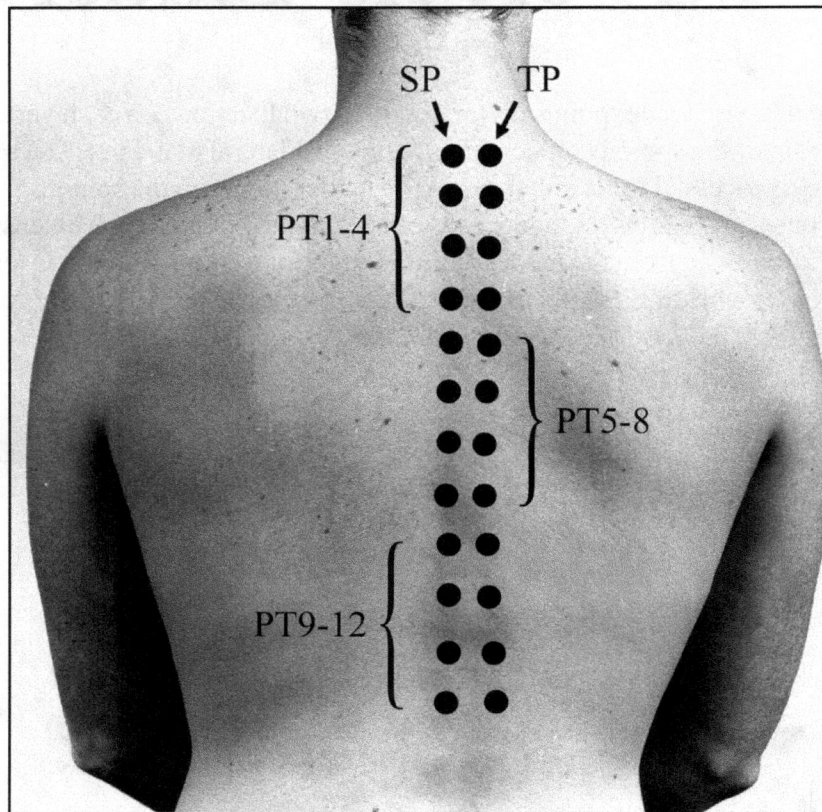

SP   TP

PT1-4

PT5-8

PT9-12

Seated Treatment for all Posterior Thoracic Points

Operator stands facing patient on opposite side of tender point. Patient sitting with head on crossed forearms leaning forward onto operator's raised knee, with head sidebent and rotated away from tender point (head rotation away induces relative torso rotation towards tender point.)

Extension.
Sidebend- away.
Rotate- toward.

E	████████
Sa	████████
Ra	████████

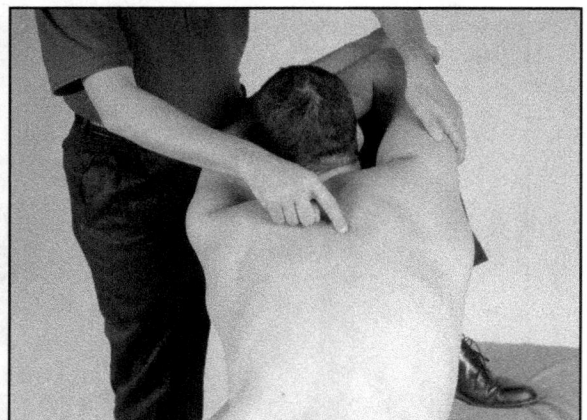

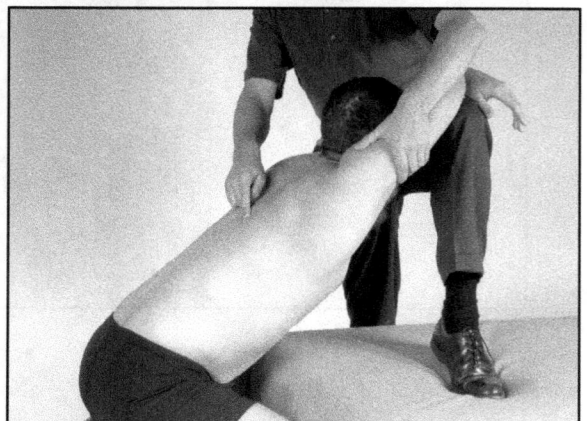

Prone Treatment for all Posterior Thoracic Points

Patient prone. Arm on the same side as tender point alongside of head on pillow for rotation and extension. Opposite arm at side. Raise arm on sore side by grasping arm above elbow. Pull arm cephalad, slightly raising for more rotation if needed. Sidebend and rotate head away from sore side especially for the upper thoracic points. For lower thoracic and lumbar points, it is often helpful to have patient simultaneously flex opposite hip and knee (see picture).
Extension-slight. More for the lower segments.
Sidebend-away. Sidebending is the major force.
Rotate- toward.

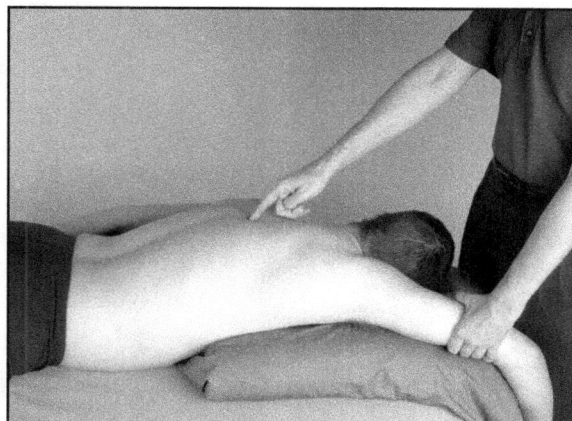

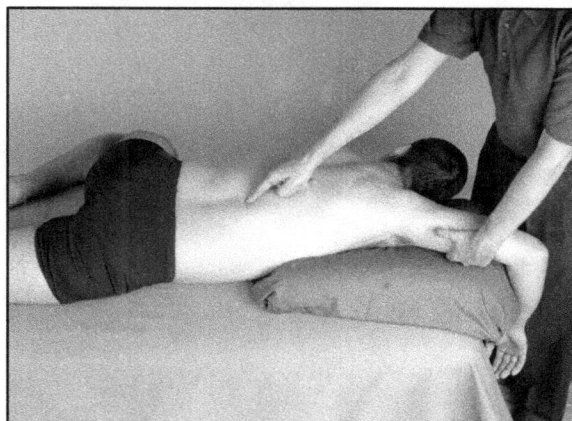

Alternate Prone Treatment for Upper Thoracic Points

Patient prone with operator at head of table holding patients chin with one hand inducing extension at level of tender point. For spinous process points little or no rotation or sidebending is needed. For transverse process points more rotation and sidebending is needed and can be introduced through patient's head. Rotation of the head <u>away</u> from the tender point will induce thoracic rotation <u>towards</u> tender point.

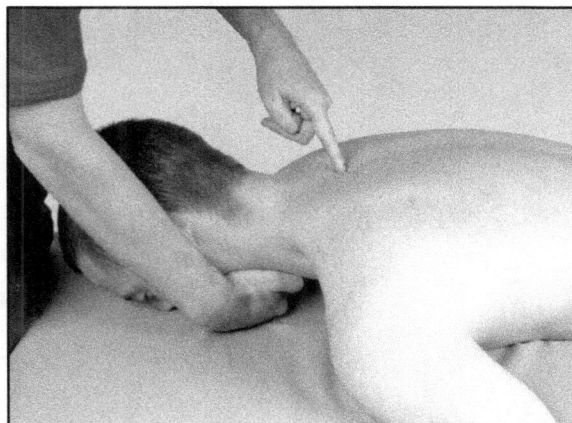

<u>**Notes**</u>

Anterior (Depressed) Rib Tender Points

Most of the anterior rib tender points are located along the anterior axillary line. The first and second anterior rib tender points are located closer to the midline. The anterior rib tender points are treated by further depressing the affected rib to exaggerate the dysfunction. When treating anterior rib tender points, additional sidebending can be induced by having the patient place both legs on the table with their feet on the same side of the table as the tender point. Have the patient take a few deep breaths to help them relax into the treatment position.

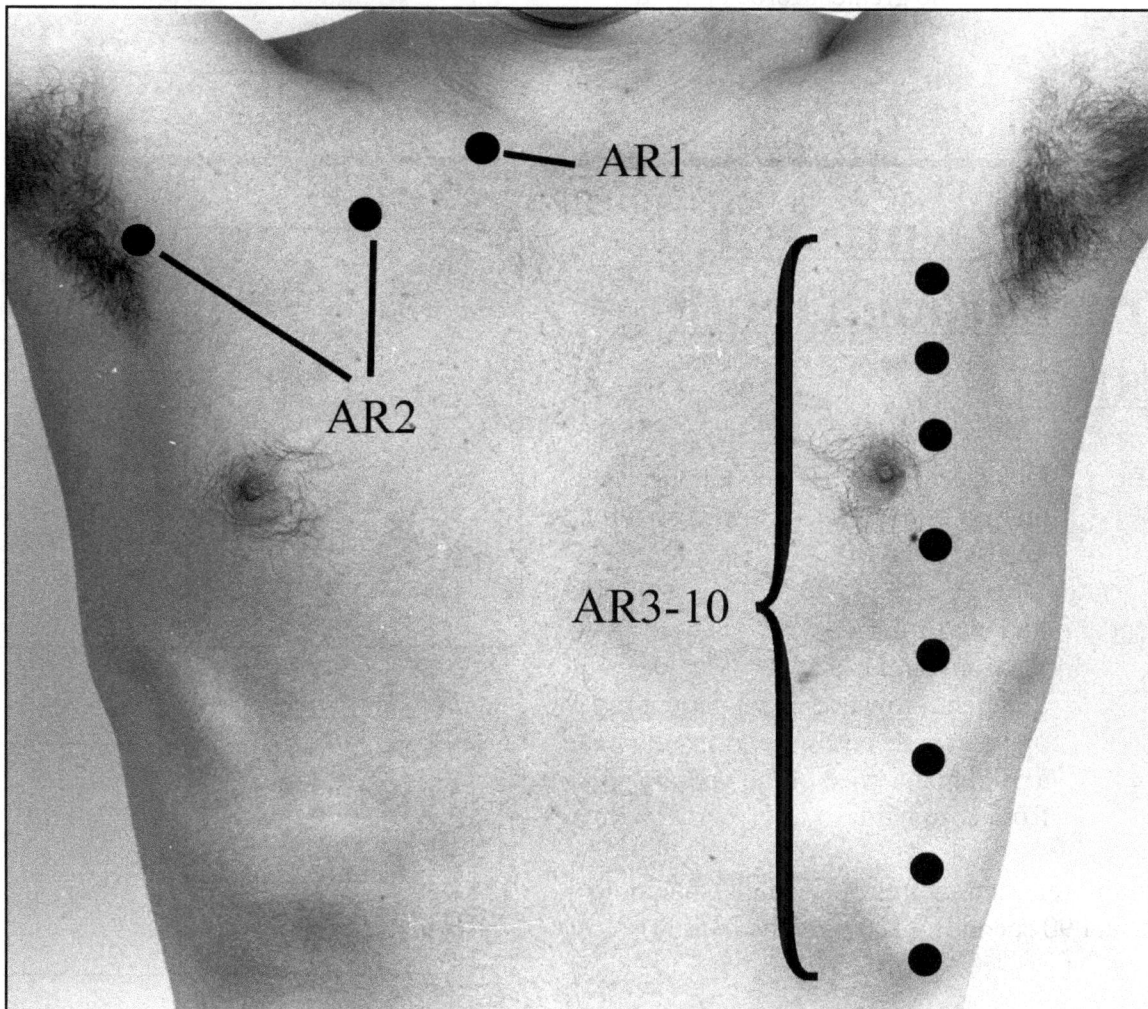

AR1-2 (Depressed First and Second Ribs)

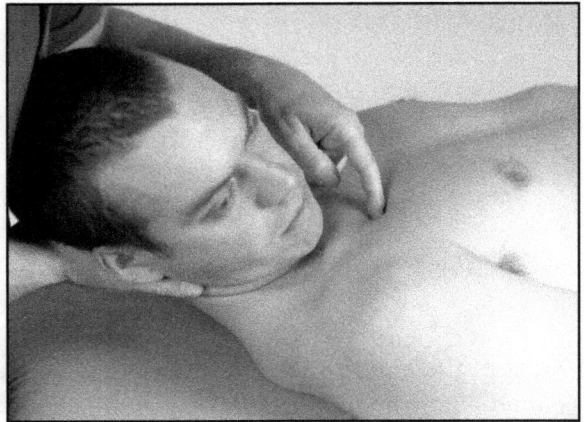

Tender Pts.   AR1- On the first costal cartilage beneath the clavicle adjacent to the sternum.

AR2- #1: 5-7 cm lateral to midline on second rib, in midclavicular line

#2: High in medial axilla.

Treatment   Patient Supine.
Flexion- slight.
Rotate- toward markedly.
Sidebend- toward the sore side.
This is the greatest force applied

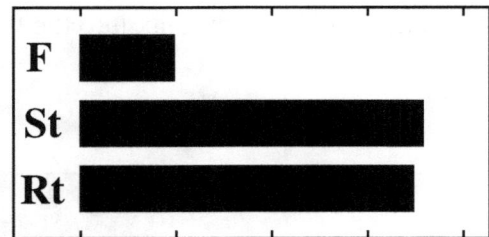

AR3-10 (Depressed Third ThroughTenth Ribs)

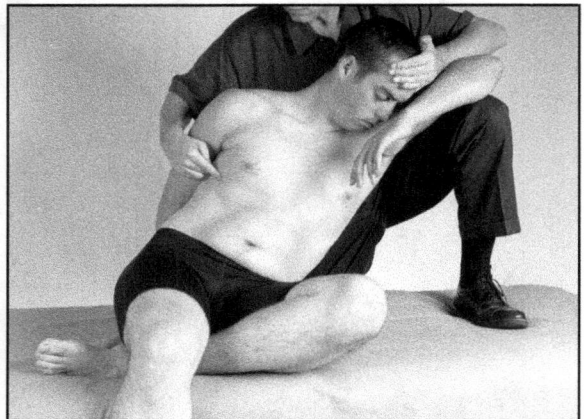

Tender Pt.   On anterior axillary line (about margin of pectoralis) at corresponding levels.

Treatment   Patient Sitting.
Flexion- slight.
Sidebend- toward. Lean patient to opposite side and support his opposite axilla on the knee of the operator.
Rotate- toward.

Tender point release requires 30 seconds, then hold for the usual 90 seconds. (120 seconds in total)

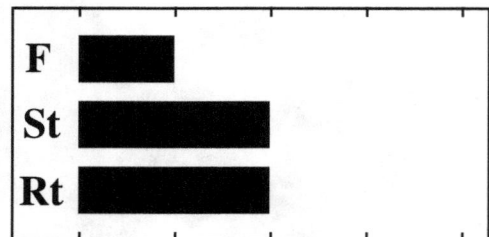

28

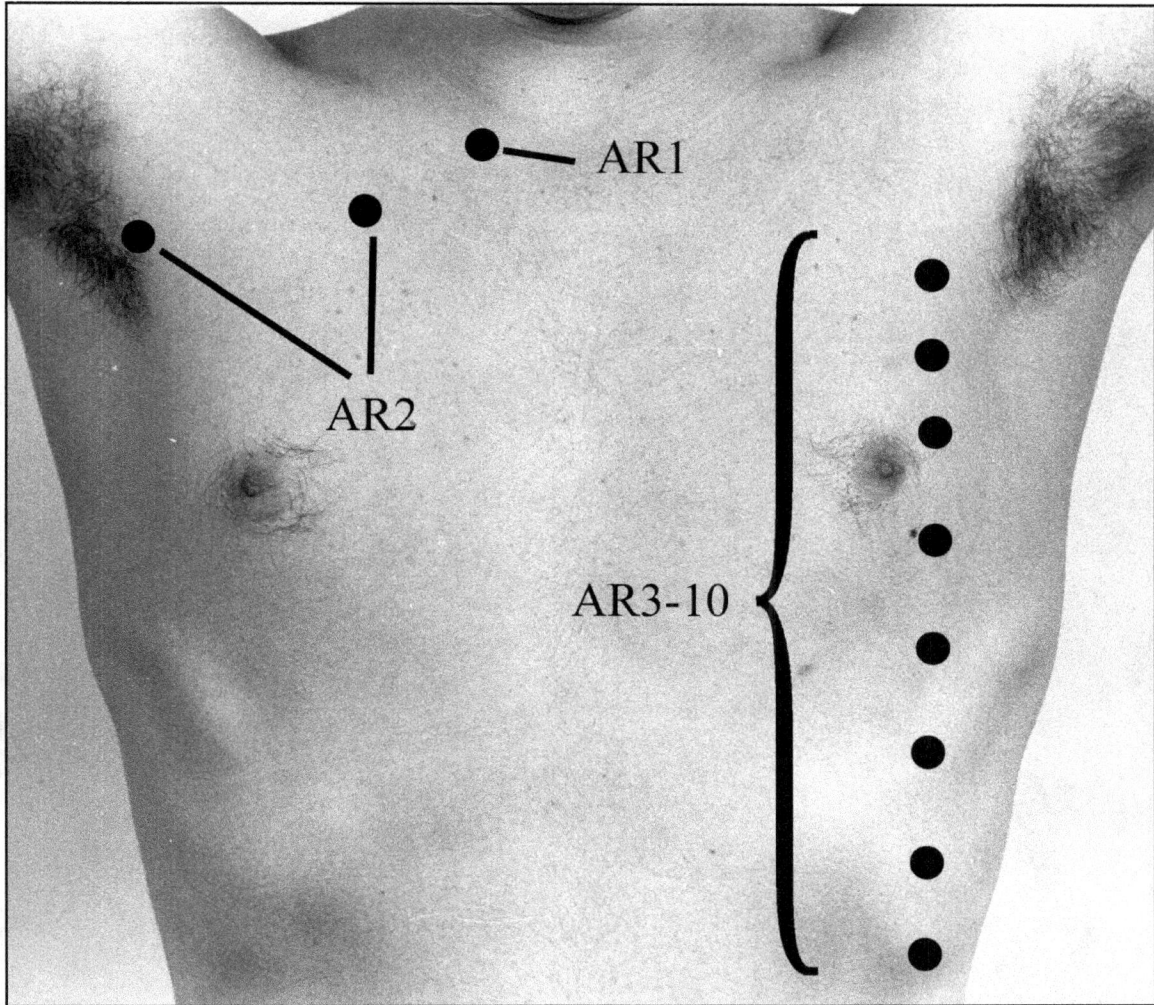

Anterior Rib Tender Points

Posterior (Elevated) Rib Tender Points

The posterior tender points are located on the rib angles and are treated by further elevating the affected rib. When treating posterior rib tender points, further sidebending can be induced by having the patient place both legs on the table with their feet on the side of the table opposite the tender point. Have the patient take a few deep breaths to help them relax into the treatment position.

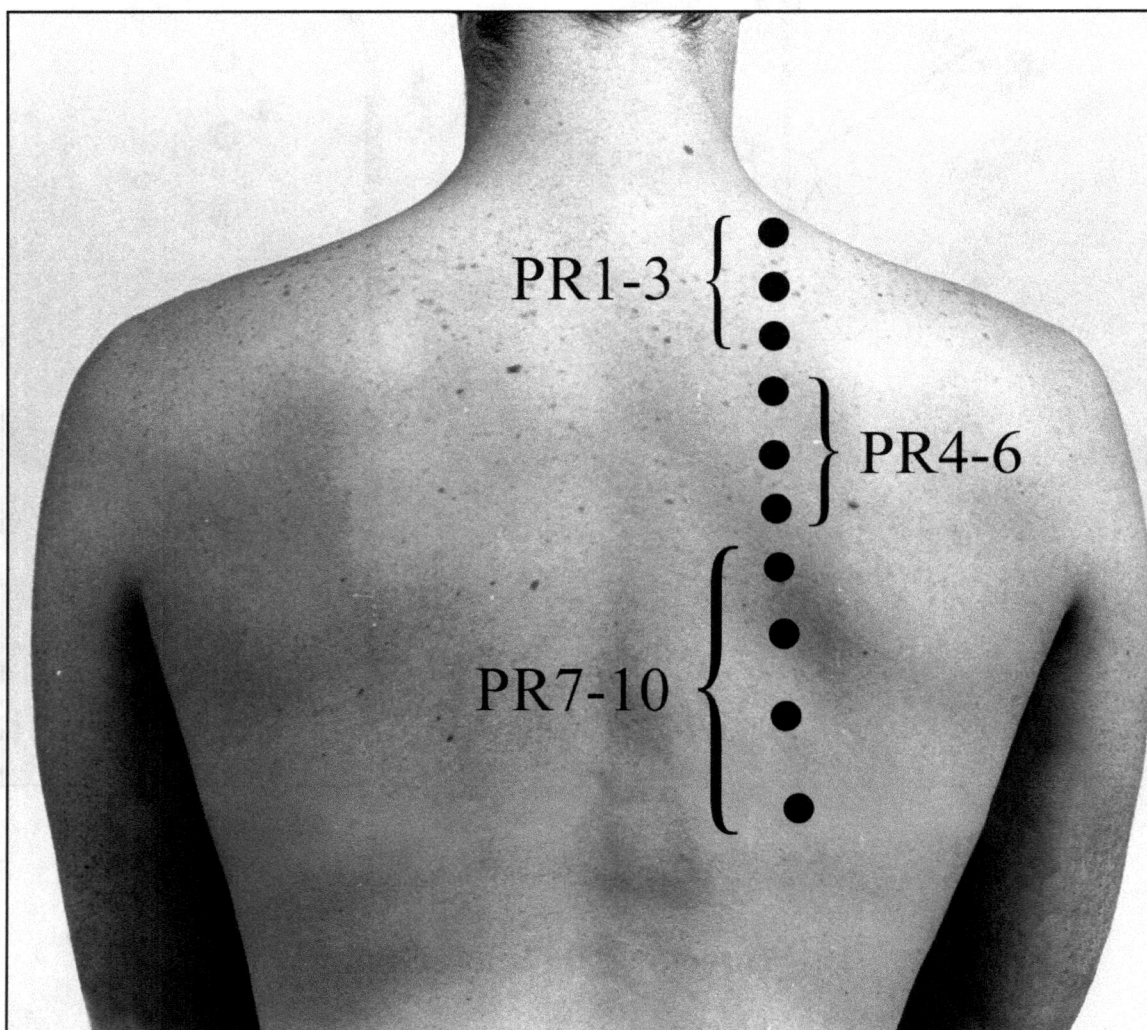

PR1-3

PR4-6

PR7-10

PR1 (Elevated First Rib)

Tender Pt.   Beneath margin of trapezius at side of neck at point that is especially tender.

Treatment   Patient sitting. Opposite axilla over operator's thigh. Lean patient mildly toward opposite side. Hold position for an extra 30 seconds.
Extension- mild.
Sidebend- usually away with head raising first rib
Rotate- toward mildly using head which induces first rib rotation in same direction.

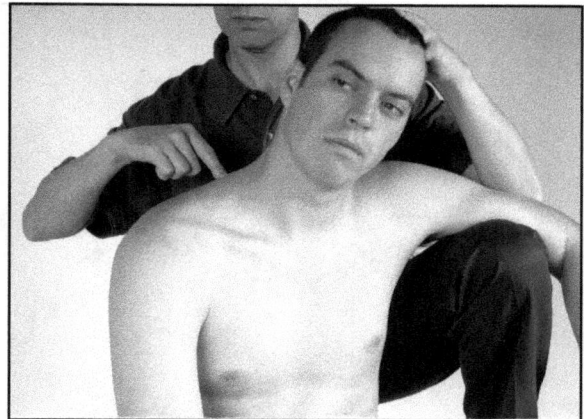

E	▮▮
Sa	▮▮▮
Rt	▮▮

PR2-10 (Elevated Second Through Tenth Ribs)

Tender Pts.   Posteriorly at angle of ribs on superior surface. Move scapula laterally to palpate by crossing arm over chest.

Treatment   Patient Sitting. Lean patient toward dysfunction and rest axilla of affected side on operator's thigh. Suspend opposite arm behind body. Patient's ipsilateral foot is placed on table under patient's opposite thigh. Hold position for an extra 30 seconds.
Sidebend- away.
Rotate- thorax away. Turning thorax with arm off table accentuates rotation of rib.(Slight head rotation towards tender point will cause further rotation away for 2nd-10th ribs)

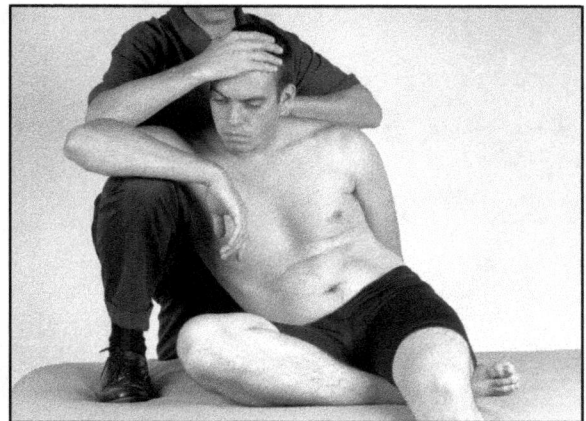

Sa	▮▮▮
Ra	▮▮▮

<u>Notes</u>

Anterior Lumbar and Pelvic Tender Points

The anterior lumbar spine tender points are mostly located around the rim of the pelvis. They can be found in association with the anterior superior or inferior iliac spines and on the anterior surface of the pubic bone. Treatment incorporates movements of the patient's legs to induce flexion, rotation and sidebending. Note rotation of the patient's legs together in one direction introduces rotation of the spine in the opposite direction. Sidebending of the pelvis in one direction induces concavity of the spine on the opposite side (low pelvis left induces right sidebent spine).

There are several anterior points useful for diagnosis and treatment of pelvic somatic dysfunction. The anterior points require flexion and rotation toward the tender point of varying amounts.

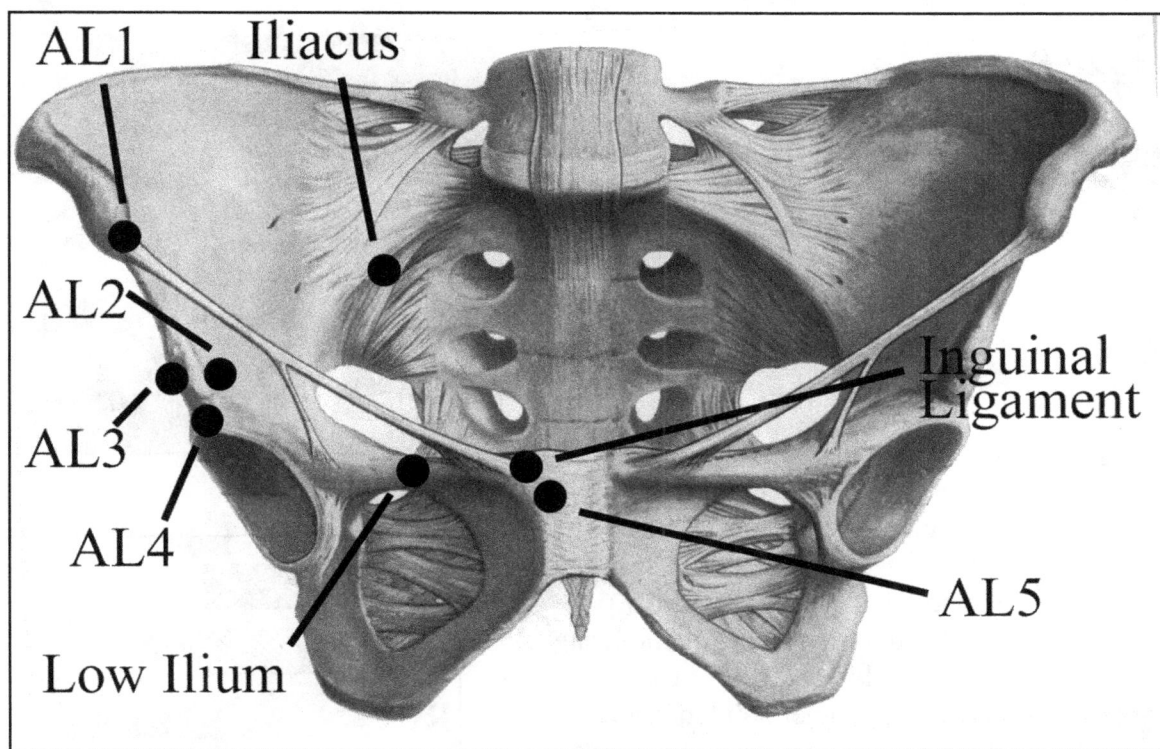

AL1

Tender Pt.   Anterior superior iliac spine.
             Approach medially, ¾" deep.

Treatment   Patient supine. Operator stands on the
             same side as the dysfunction inducing
             flexion to the level of the dysfunction.
             Place several pillows under hips of the
             patient to obtain additional flexion of
             pelvis on lumbar spine. Rest patient's
             flexed legs on doctor's thigh.
             Flexion- moderate to marked
             Sidebend- toward (patient's opposite
               hip inferior)
             Rotate- away (patient's knees towards
               operator, torso rotates relatively
               away)

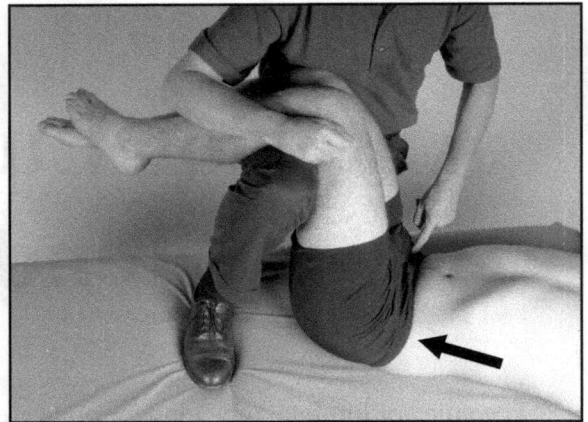

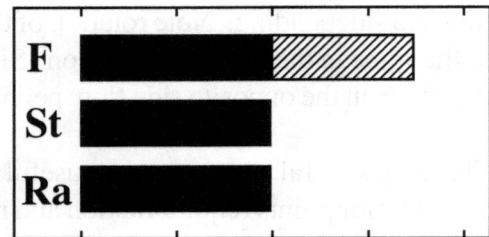

F		
St		
Ra		

AL2-4

Tender Pts. AL2- Medial surface of anterior iliac
               spine.
             AL3- Lateral surface of anterior iliac
               spine.
             AL4- Inferior to anterior inferior iliac
               spine. Slightly below AL3 tender
               point.

Treatment   Patient Supine. Operator stands on
             opposite side of the dysfunction. Note:
             motions introduced are relative to the
             spinal level being treated.
             Flexion- patient's legs flexed 90°
             Sidebend- away slightly to moderate,
               more for lower levels (patient's hip
               on side of tender point inferior)
             Rotate- toward markedly (patient's
               knees towards opearator)

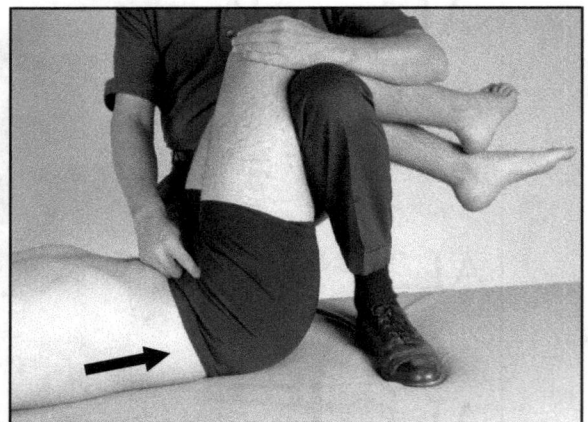

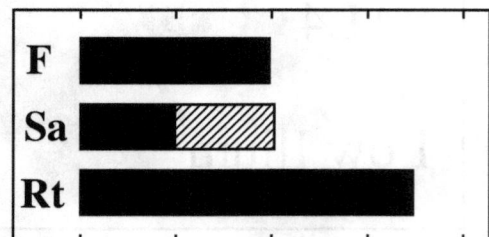

F		
Sa		
Rt		

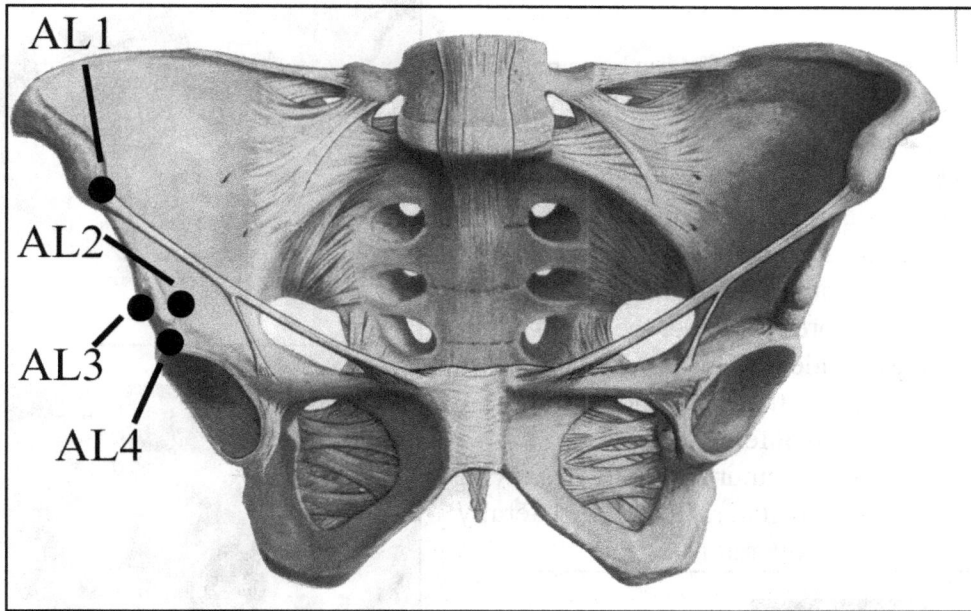

Tender points for AL1-4

AL5

<u>Tender Pt.</u> Anterior superior aspect of pubic bone. 1 cm lateral to symphysis pubis.

<u>Treatment</u> Patient Supine. Operator stands on same side as tender point.
Flexion- marked
Sidebend- away (patient's opposite hip moves superiorly)
Rotate- away (patient's knees towards operator)

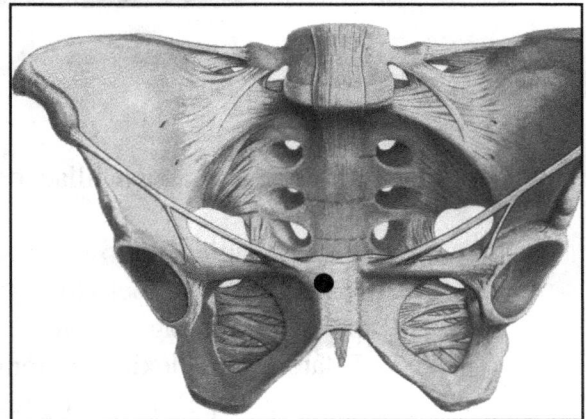

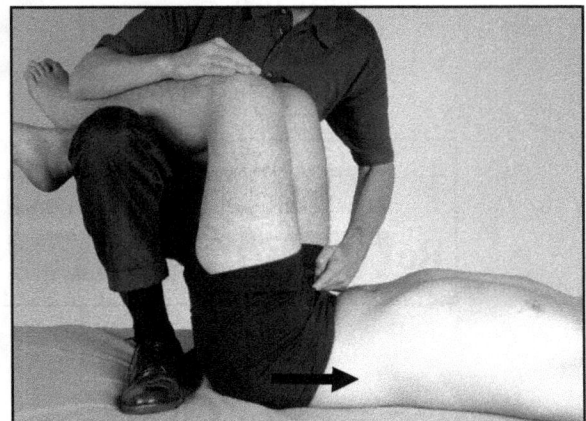

F	
Sa	
Ra	

Inguinal Ligament

Tender Pt.   Superior surface of pubic bone near the inguinal ligament attachment.

Treatment   Patient Supine. Operator stands on same side as tender point.
Flexion- Flex both legs 90° and rest on operator's thigh. Move the leg on the sore side under the opposite leg of patient. This produces crossing of the knees and thighs.
Adduction- of femur.
Rotation- of femur internally by moving patient's ipsilateral lower leg laterally (towards operator)

F	████████
Ad	████████
Ri	████████

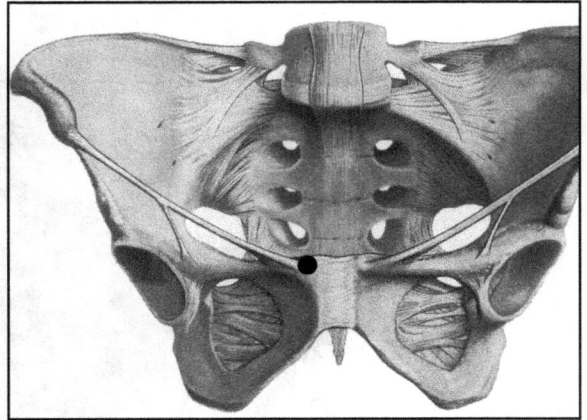

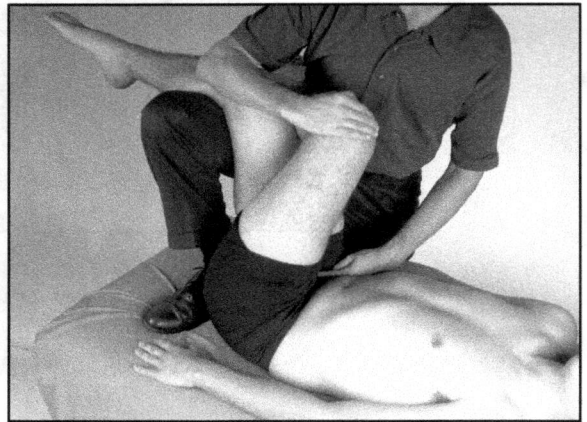

Iliacus

Tender Pt.   Anterior and deep in illiac fossa.

Treatment   Patient Supine. Pillow can be placed under buttocks to raise pelvis, increasing flexion.
Bilateral Hip Flexion- extreme
Bilateral Hip Rotation- extreme external

F	████████████
Re	████████████

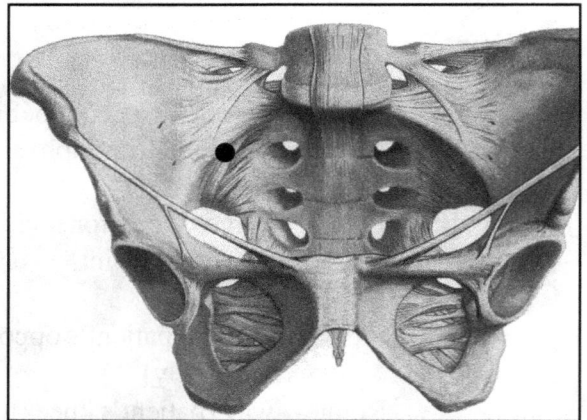

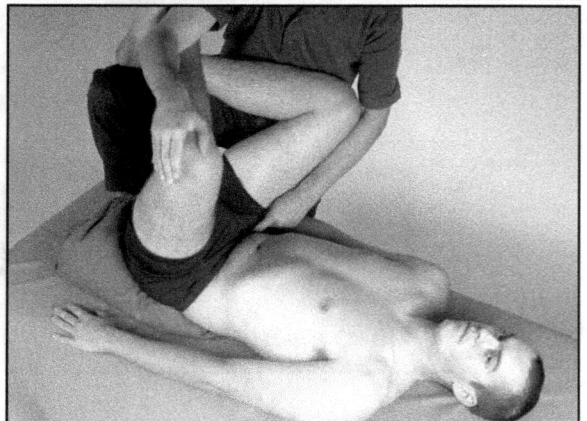

Low Ilium (Sacroilliac)

Tender Pt.   Lateral ramus of pubic bone on anterior surface.

Treatment   Patient Supine.
Flexion-of thigh on sore side, usually to 90°
Abduction- sometimes needed
Sidebend- none.
Rotate- none.

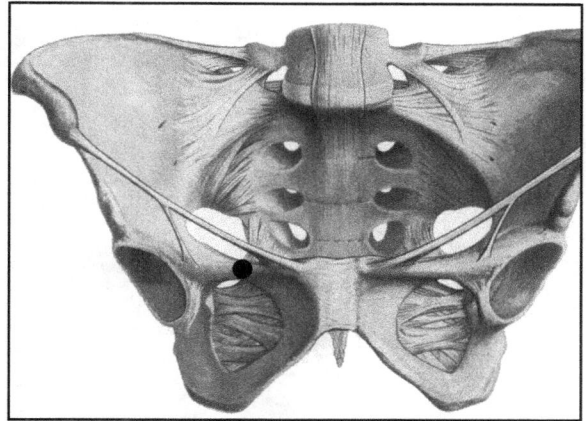

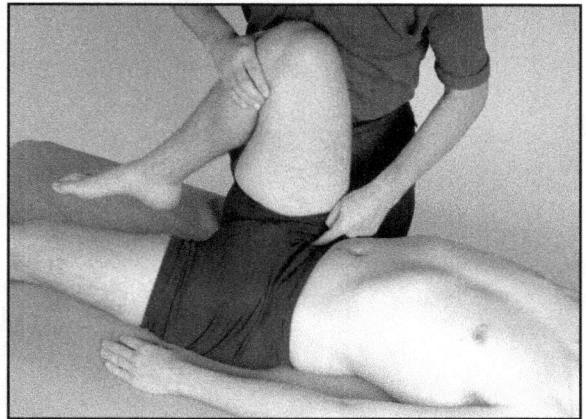

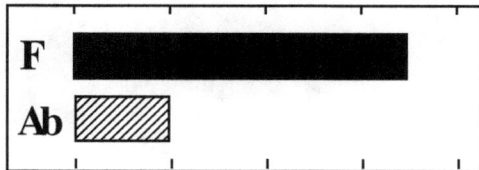

Notes

Posterior Lumbar and Pelvic Tender Points

Posterior lumbar tender points are found mostly along the spinous processes (SP) in the same places as in the thoracic spine, although tender points found on the tips of the transverse processes (TP) are approached by pressing anteromedially at about a forty five degree angle due to the increased volume of myofascial tissue to palpate through. These tender points typically require extension and rotation away from the tender point

Tender points are also associated with the muscle attachments and muscles of the sacrum and pelvis. Extension is the predominant motion associated with the posterior tender points, although various amounts of abduction, adduction and rotation may also be needed.

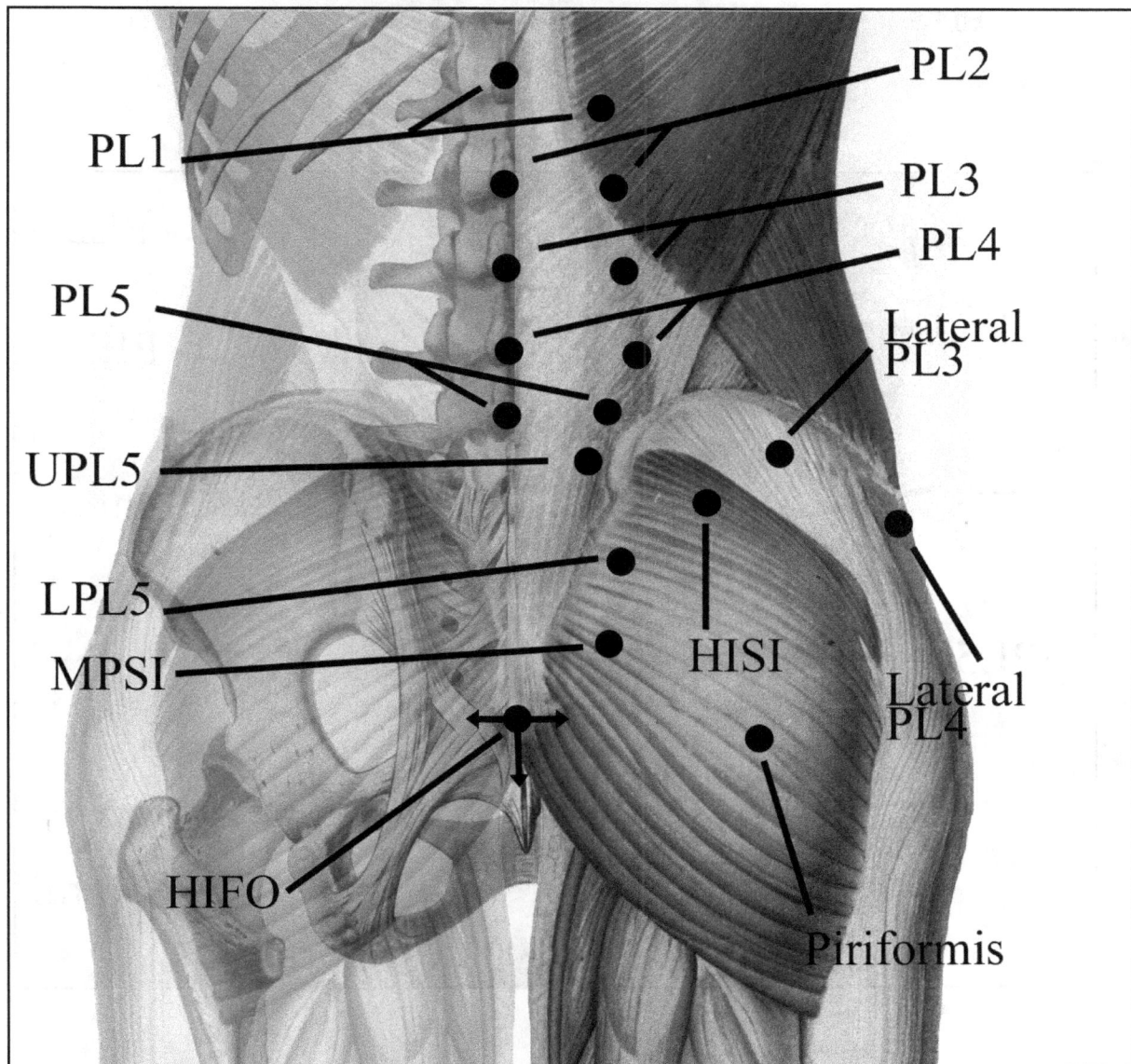

PL1-5 (SP) & (TP), PL3-4 Lateral, UPL5 (Upper Pole)

Tender Pts. **PL 1-5:** Lateral to spinous processes (SP) or on tip of transverse processes (TP) of corresponding vertebrae.

Lat L3: In superior gluteal region halfway between PSIS (post. sup. iliac spine) and lateral iliac crest, about 1 cm superior to PSIS.

Lat L4: On lateral aspect of iliac crest in superior gluteal region at about same level as PSIS.

UPL5: Just medial and superior to PSIS.

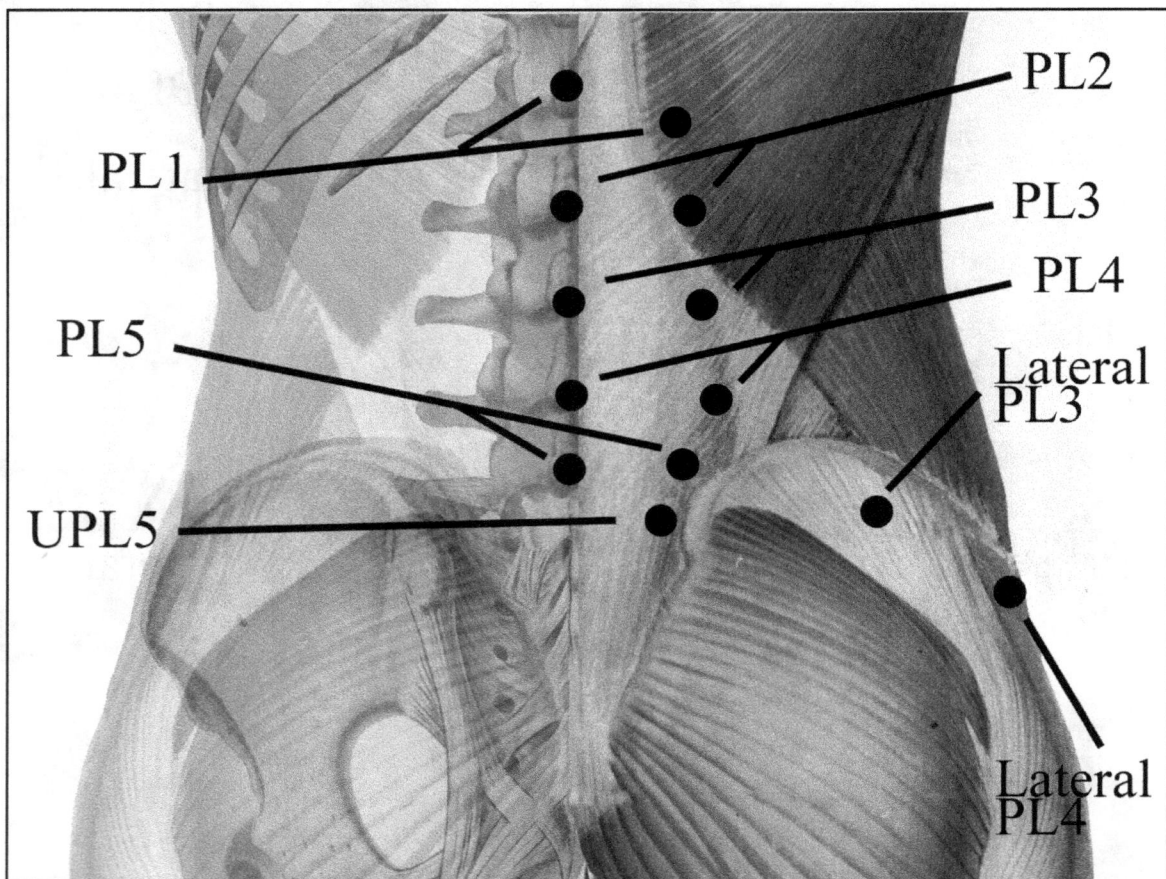

Treatment   Patient prone, Operator on opposite
side. Operator lifts patient's legs
together (SP) or contralateral leg
(TP) over operator's knee holding
patient's leg above knee.
Extension- moderate to marked, more
for upper lumbars
Sidebend- away, move patient's leg(s)
towards operator.
Rotate- towards, raise leg up on side
opposite operator.

Note: Because of marked extension, rotation goes
above level of tender point. It is therefore in the same
direction as leg rotation.

Treatment position for SP tender points

Treatment position for TP tender points

Alternate treatment for Lat L3-L4, UPL5
Operator stands on same side as dysfunction and lifts patient's leg over operator's
knee holding patient's leg above the knee.

Alternate treatment for Lat L3-L4, UPL5

LPL5 (Lower Pole)

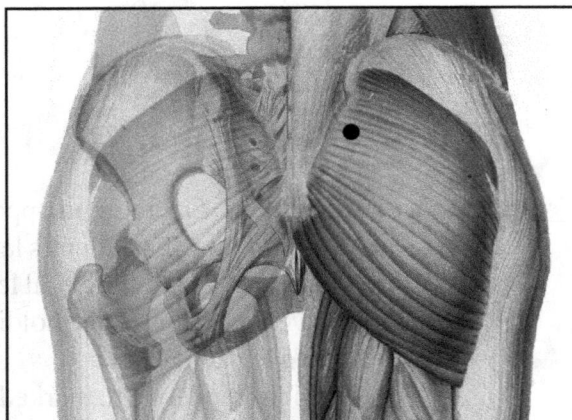

Tender Pt.   1 cm below PSIS in small saddle between PSIS and PIIS. Also on spinous process of L5.

Treatment   Patient prone. Operator seated on side of dysfunction. Leg on sore side is dropped off of table resting on operator's thigh. Patient's thigh flexed 90°. Patient's pelvis is rotated away and the knee is adducted slightly.
Flexion.
Sidebend- toward.
Rotate- toward.

F	████████
St	████████
Rt	████████

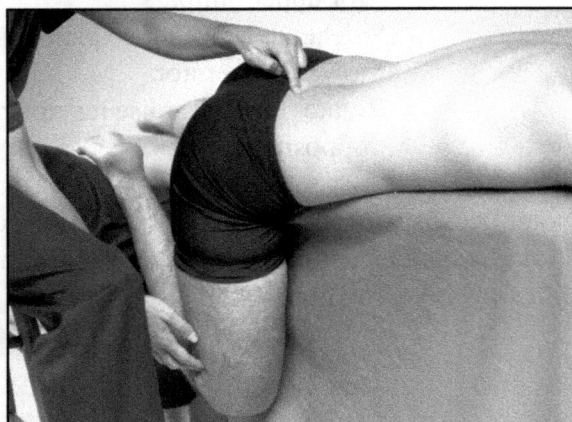

High Ilium Sacroiliac (HISI)

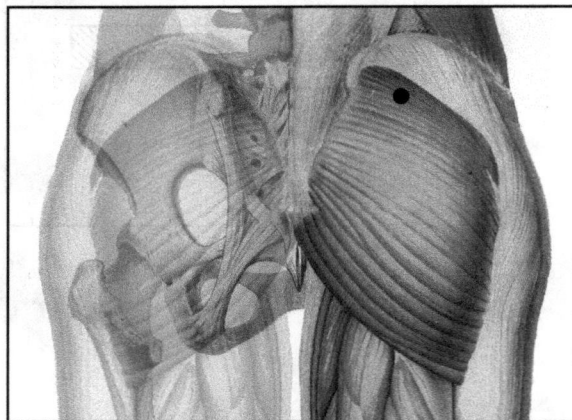

Tender Pt.   4-5 cm lateral to posterior superior iliac spine.

Treatment   Patient Supine.
Extension.
Abduction- slight.

E	████████
Ab	████

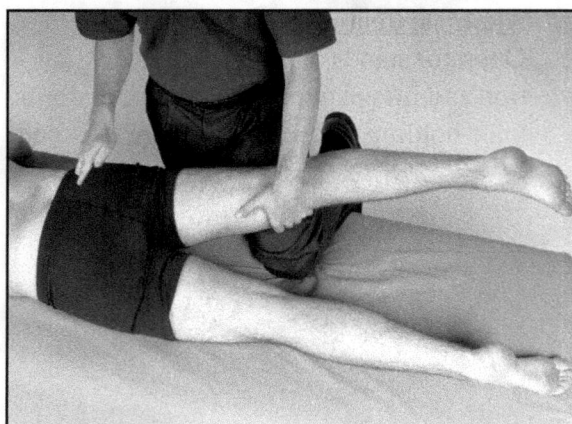

Mid-Pole Sacroilliac: Ilium Flare In- Superiorly (MPSI)

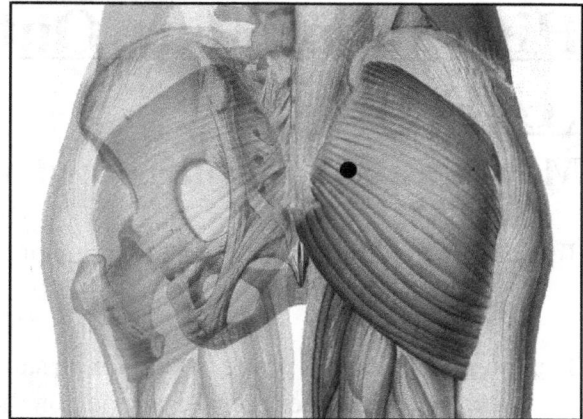

Tender Pt.   3-4 cm caudad to posterior superior iliac spine in muscle depression lateral to sacrum. Approach the tender point from the side.

Treatment   Patient prone.
Flexion- slight of hip and knee.
Abduction- of leg, is major component
Rotation- external of hip

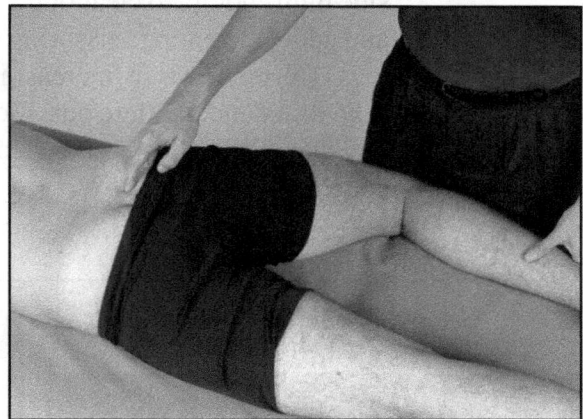

F	███
Ab	████
Re	████

Piriformis (PIR)

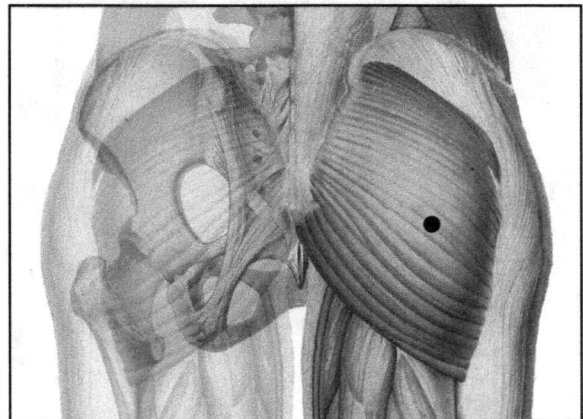

Tender Pt.   In piriformis muscle 8-9 cm medial to and slightly cephalad to the greater trochanter.

Treatment   Similar to PL5.
Patient prone. Operator is seated on side of tender point. Patient's leg is suspended off table with patient's leg resting on operator's thigh.
Flexion- hip 135°.
Abduct- knee slightly
Rotation- variable internal or external

F	████
Ab	██
Ri/Re	██▨

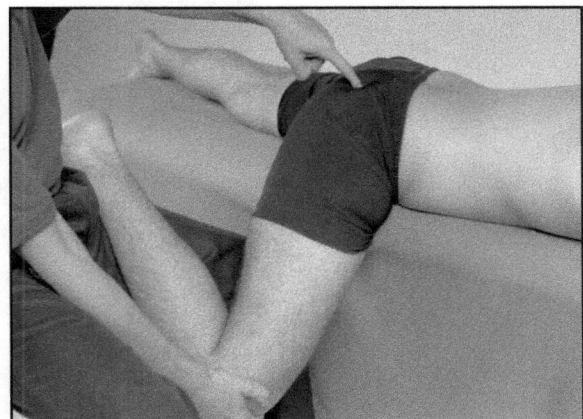

43

High Ilium Flare Out (HIFO)

May be associated with coccydynia

Tender Pts.   At sacrococcygeal junction or on coccyx.

Treatment   Patient prone. Operator on same side as tender point. Raise leg on the sore side high enough to clear opposite leg and <u>adduct</u>, creating scissoring of the legs. Correction is by increasing the high ilium and the flare out. Occasionally the opposite leg is extended and adducted.

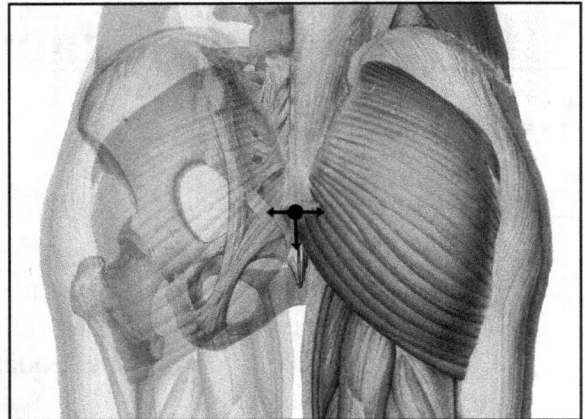

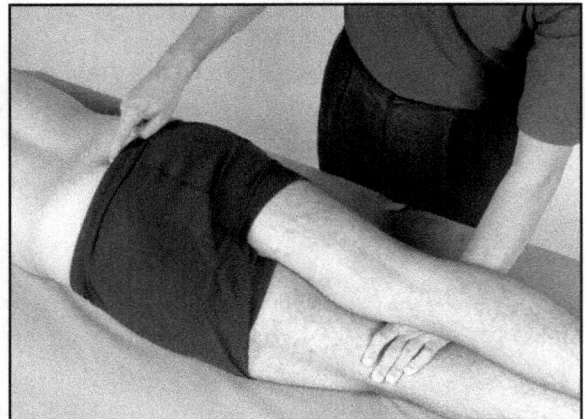

Axillary Region
Tender Points

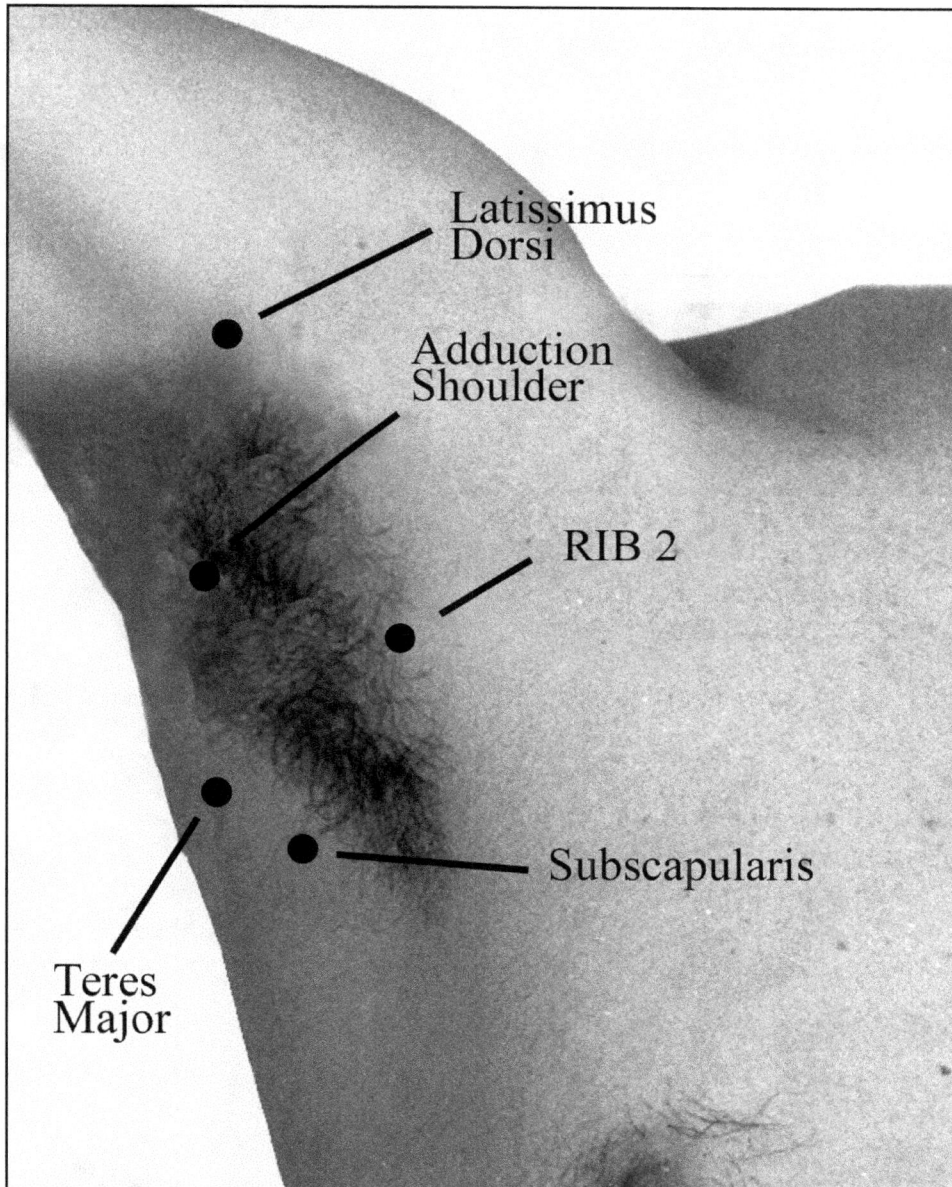

Latissimus
Dorsi

Adduction
Shoulder

RIB 2

Subscapularis

Teres
Major

Rib 2 (R2)

Tender Pt.   Deep in the axilla on the midaxillary line.

Treatment   Patient supine, operator on same side as tender point
Abduction- marked of shoulder.
Traction- gentle.

The scapula, clavicle and AC joint can be stabilized by compressing the shoulder medial to glenohumeral joint.

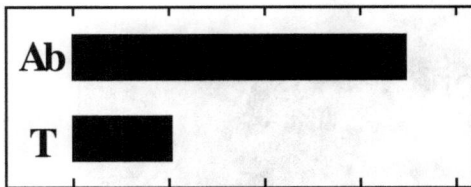

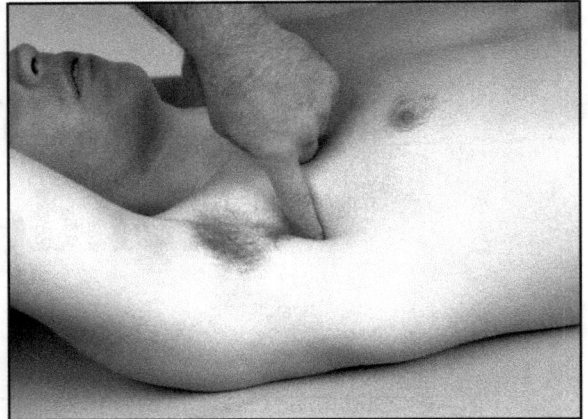

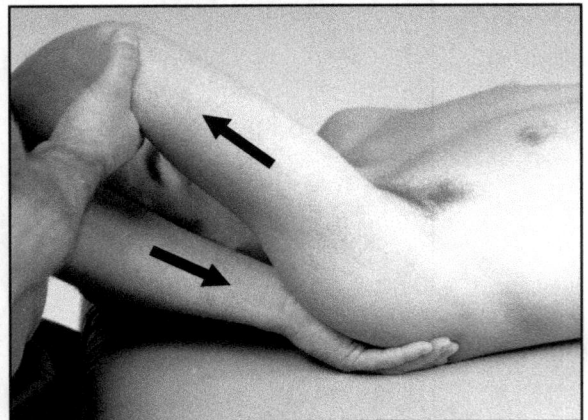

Ab	███████████
T	███

Subscapularis (SUB)

Tender Pt.   On the anterior surface of the scapula, in the posterior axillary fold.

Treatment   Patient supine, shoulder on table.
Extension- 30°– 40°
Rotation- internal
Abduction- slight
Traction- usually marked, 3kg, verbally ask patient to relax their shoulder

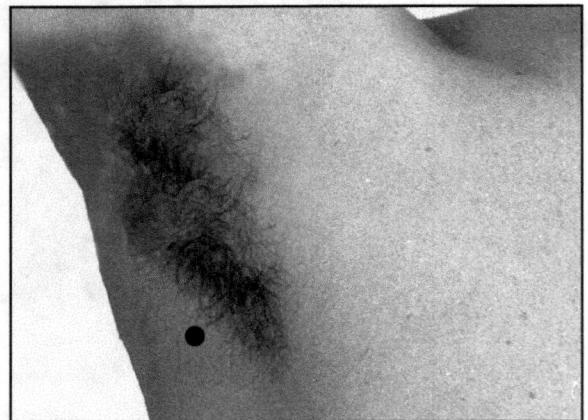

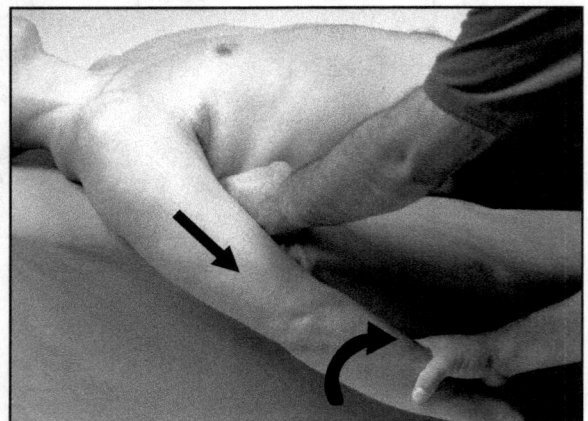

E	██████
Ri	██████
Ab	███
T	█████████

Teres Major (TM)

<u>Tender Pt.</u>   On the lateral margin of the scapula

<u>Treatment</u>   Patient supine
Extension- moderate
Abduction- slight
Rotation- marked internal

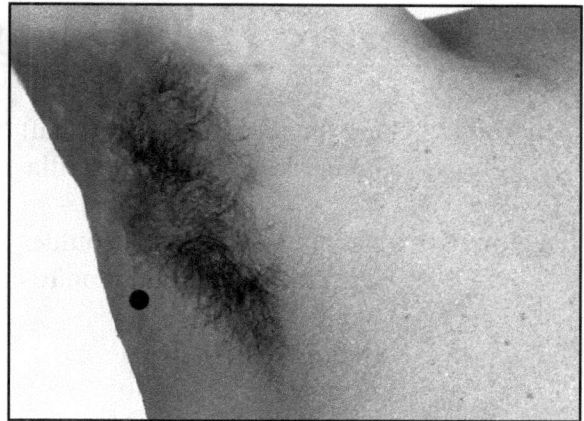

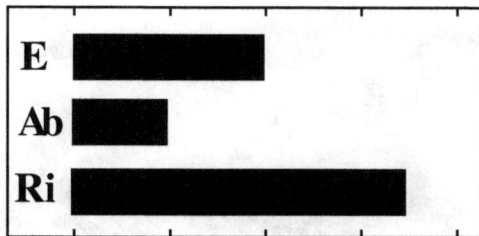

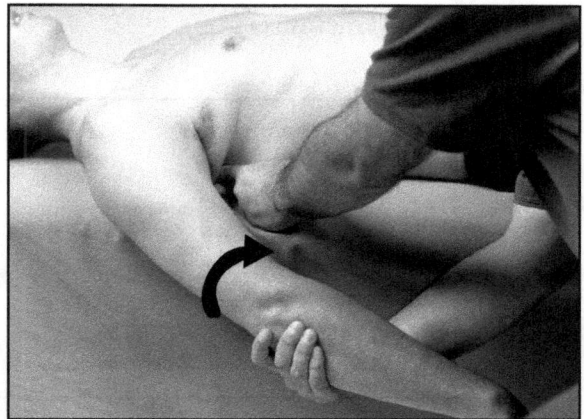

E	▬▬▬▬▬
Ab	▬▬▬
Ri	▬▬▬▬▬▬▬

Adduction Shoulder (Frozen Shoulder)

<u>Tender Pt.</u>   High in the lateral wall of the axilla. Diagnosis can be made if patient holds elbow tightly to chest and will not move it.

<u>Treatment</u>   Patient supine. Operator places one hand in patient's axilla, the other on elbow inducing hyper-adduction of shoulder.
Adduction- marked
Rotation- slight internal
Compression- slight at elbow

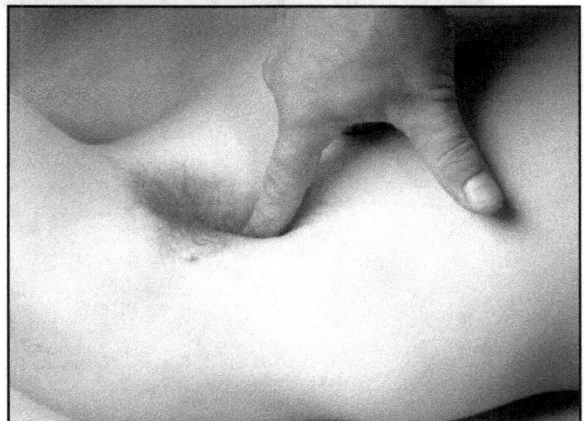

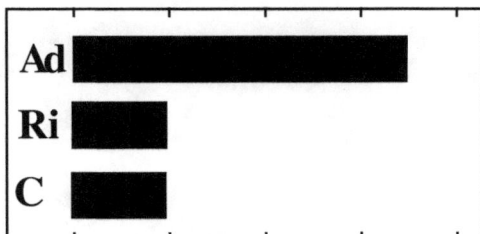

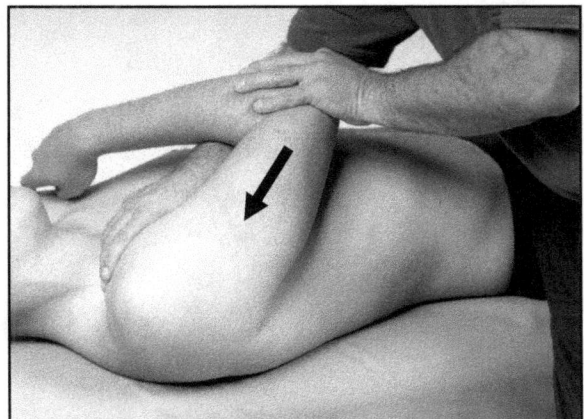

Ad	▬▬▬▬▬▬▬
Ri	▬▬▬
C	▬▬▬

Latissimus Dorsi (LD)

Tender Pt.
On the medial superior shaft of the humerus in the lateral axilla

Treatment
Patient supine with shoulder off table. Operator applies traction to arm from wrist.
Extension- 30-40°
Abduction- about 30°
Rotation- internal
Traction- strong

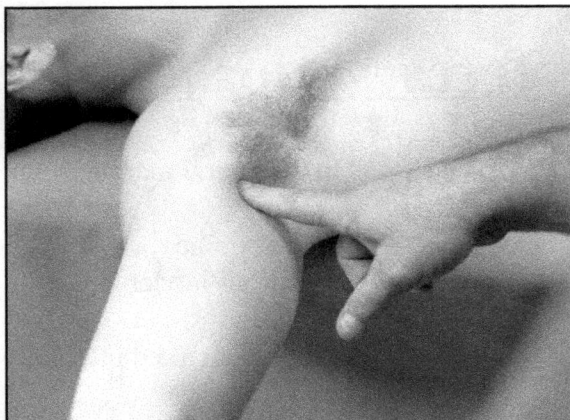

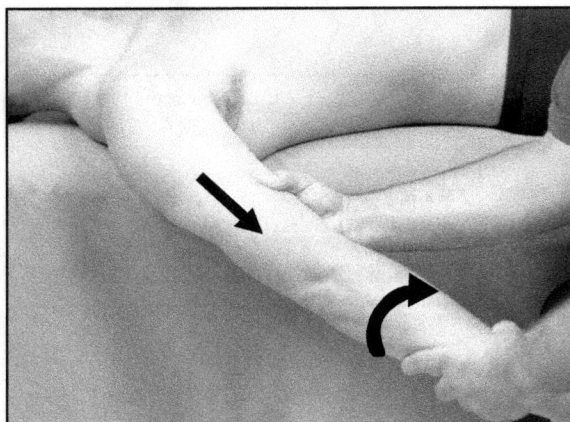

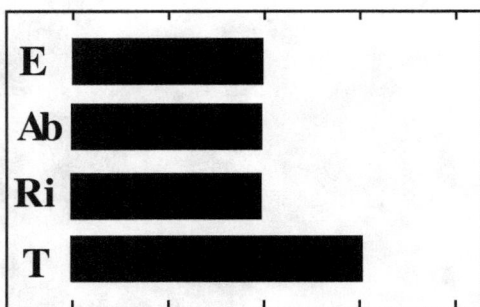

Posterior Shoulder Tender Points

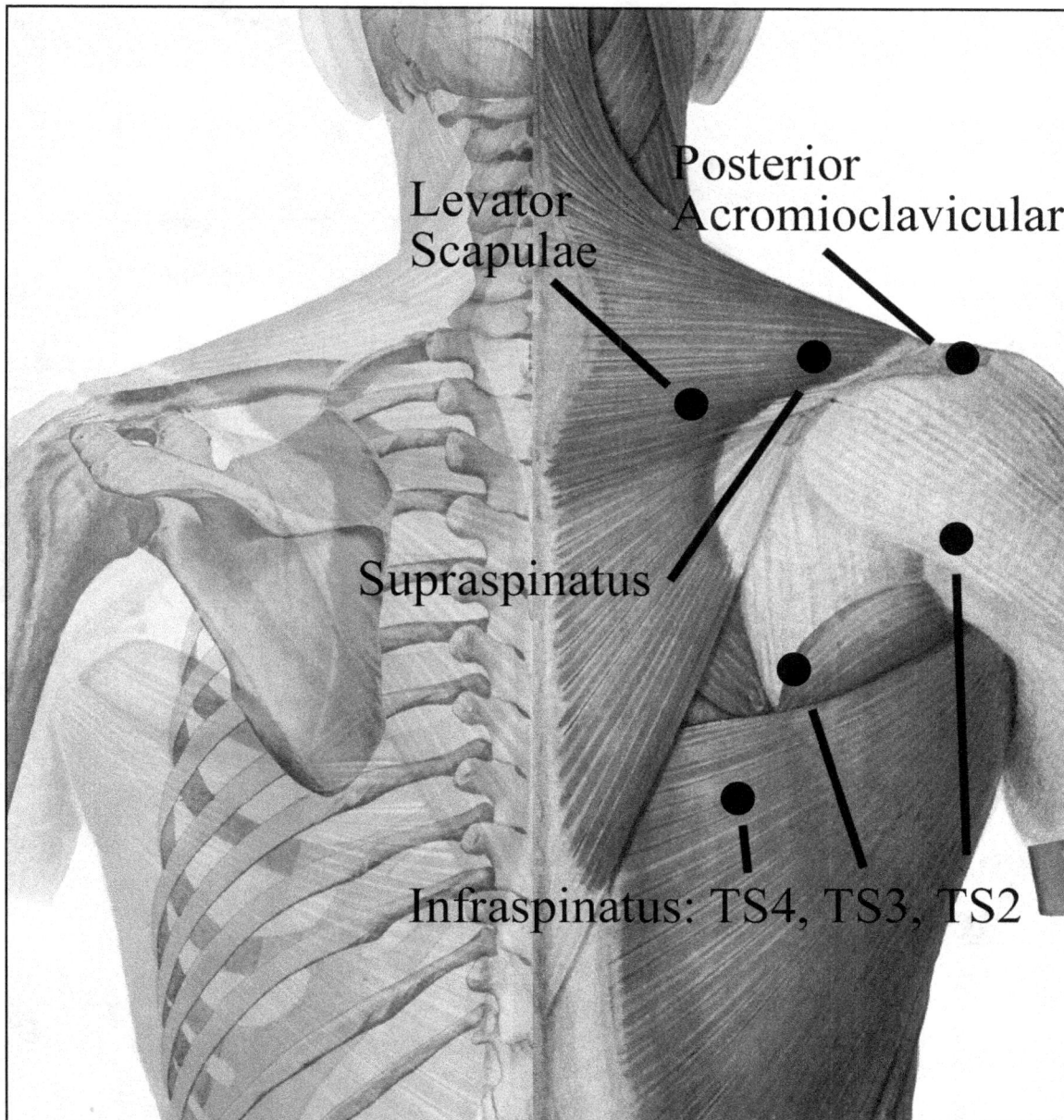

Levator Scapulae

Posterior Acromioclavicular

Supraspinatus

Infraspinatus: TS4, TS3, TS2

Supraspinatus (SPI)

<u>Tender Pt.</u>   Medial to posterior AC in
                suraspinatus fossa.

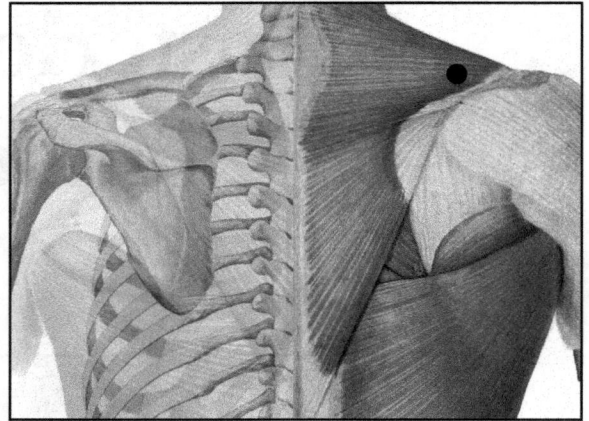

Infraspinatus- Second Thoracic Shoulder (TS2)

<u>Tender Pt.</u>   1 cm. Below lateral edge of scapular
                spine.

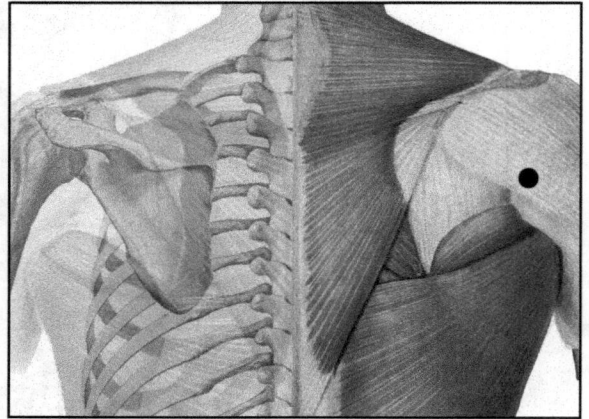

Infraspinatus- Third Thoracic Shoulder (TS3)

<u>Tender Pt.</u>   In body of infraspinatus, 7-8 cm.
                below spine of scapula and 2-3 cm.
                lateral to medial margin.

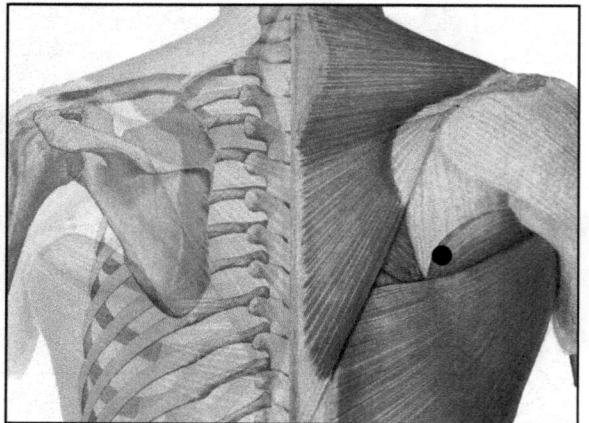

Infraspinatus- Fourth Thoracic Shoulder (TS4)

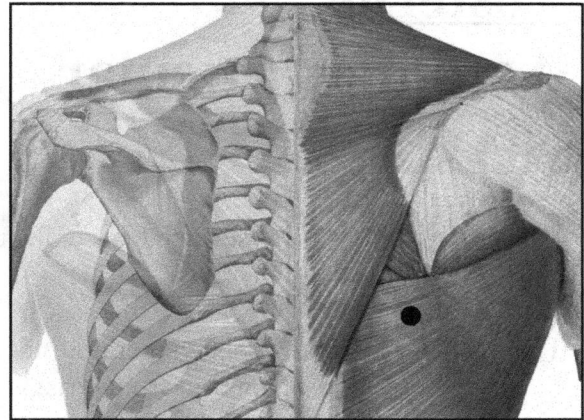

Tender Pt. In muscle mass at lower tip of scapula.

Treatment for Infraspinatus and Supraspinatus Tender Points:

Treatment Patient supine, Operator elevates patient arm over head. (Statue of Liberty)
Flexion- 90°
Rotation- variable external
Adduction- slight
Traction- mild

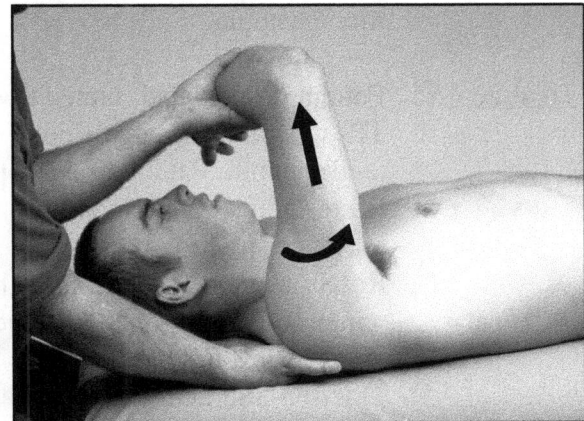

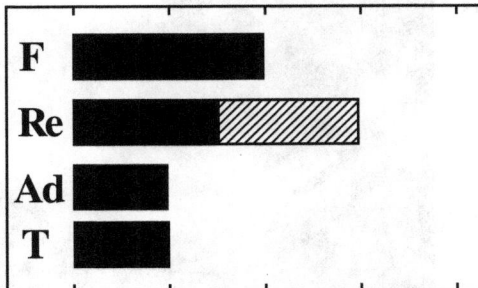

Posterior Acromioclavicular (PAC)

Tender Pt.   Posterior surface of lateral, superior acromion.

Treatment   Patient prone. Operator places traction on arm from wrist.
Extension- slight
Adduction- slight
Traction- marked

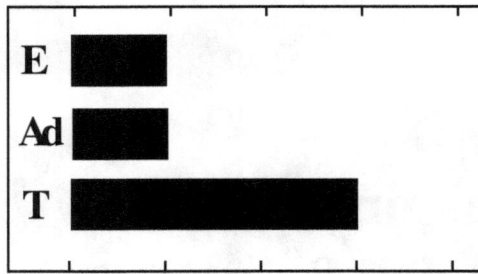

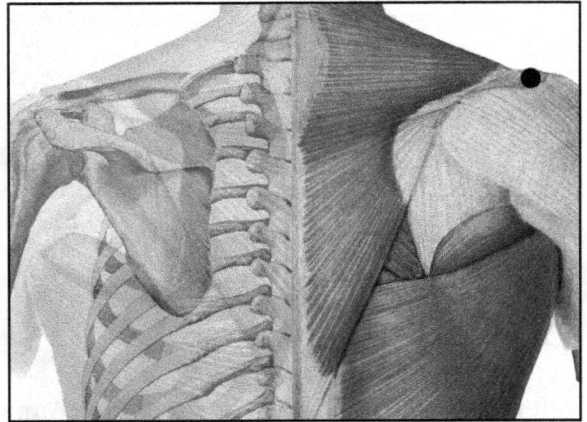

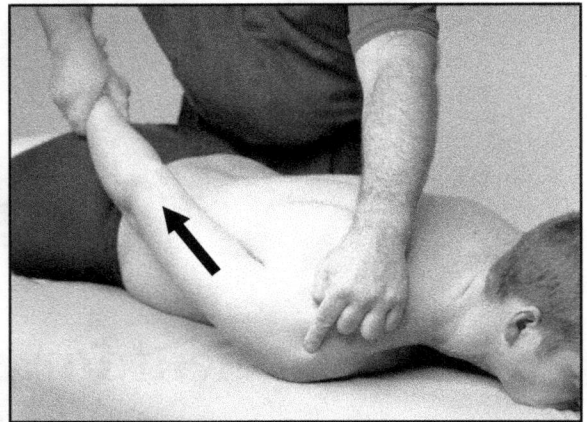

E	████
Ad	████
T	████████

Levator Scapulae (LS)

Tender Pt.   In muscle tissue on superior, medial tip of scapula.

Treatment   Patient prone, head rotated towards TP. Operator on same side of table as tender point. Patient grasps operator's leg to induce rotation of arm. Operator places traction on arm.
Rotation- moderate of arm either internally or externally (whichever is of greatest ease to patient)
Traction- marked

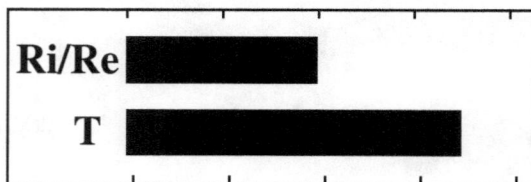

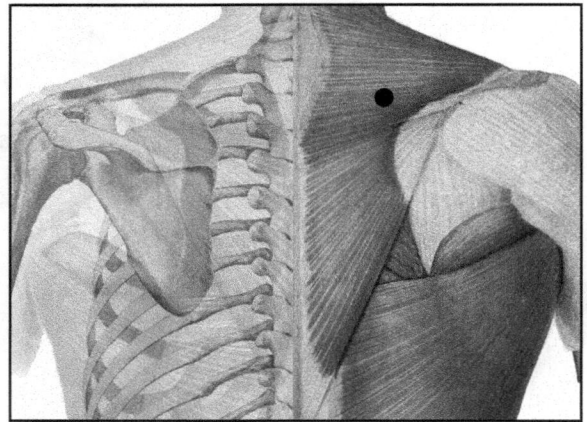

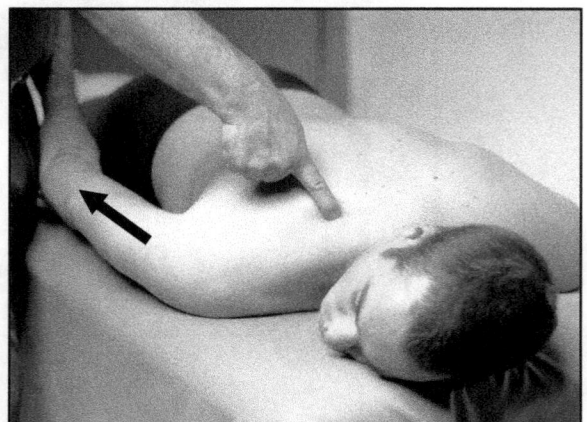

Ri/Re	█████
T	███████

Upper Extremity Tender Points

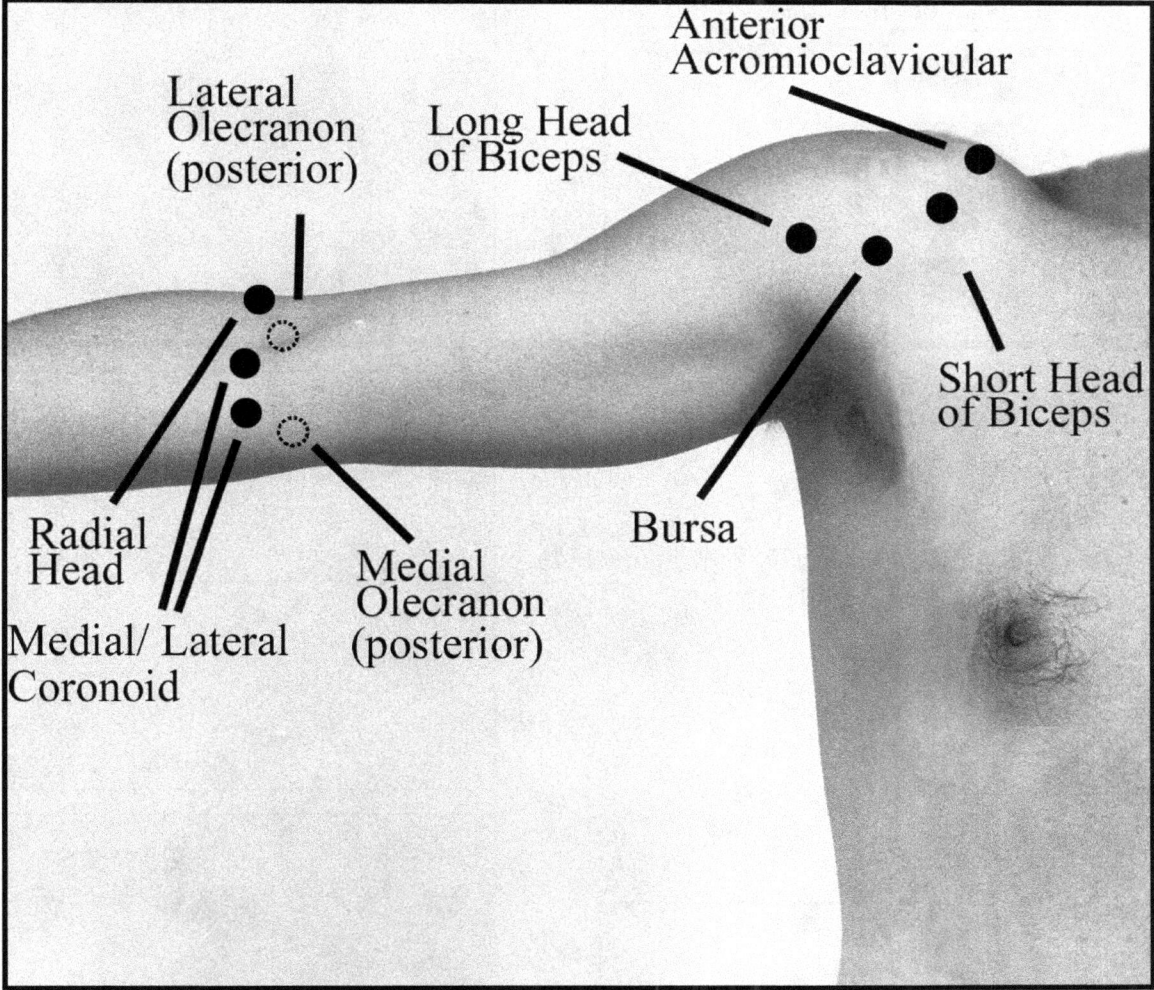

Lateral
Olecranon
(posterior)

Long Head
of Biceps

Anterior
Acromioclavicular

Short Head
of Biceps

Radial
Head

Medial/ Lateral
Coronoid

Medial
Olecranon
(posterior)

Bursa

Anterior Acromioclavicular (AAC)

Tender Pt.   Anterior surface of the distal clavicle.

Treatment   Patient supine. Operator on opposite
             side of table as tender point, applies
             traction of arm across chest and
             cephalad.
             Adduction- variable 30-50°
             Flexion- slight
             Rotation- internal
             Traction- moderate

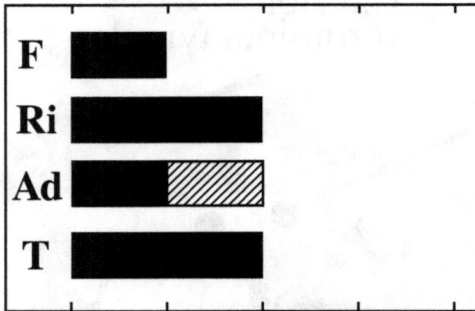

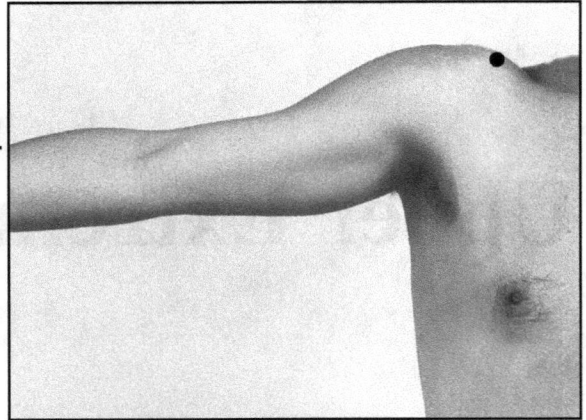

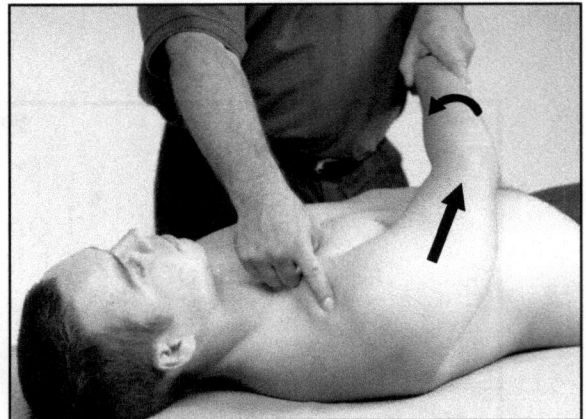

F	████	
Ri	████████	
Ad	██▨▨▨	
T	██████	

Short Head of Biceps (SHB)

Tender Pt.   Infero-lateral surface of the coracoid
             process of scapula

Treatment   Patient supine.
             Flexion- variable
             Adduction- moderate
             Rotation- usually internal

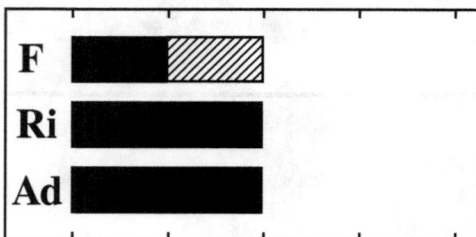

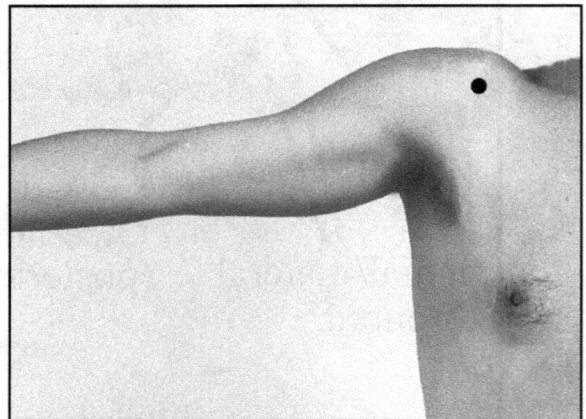

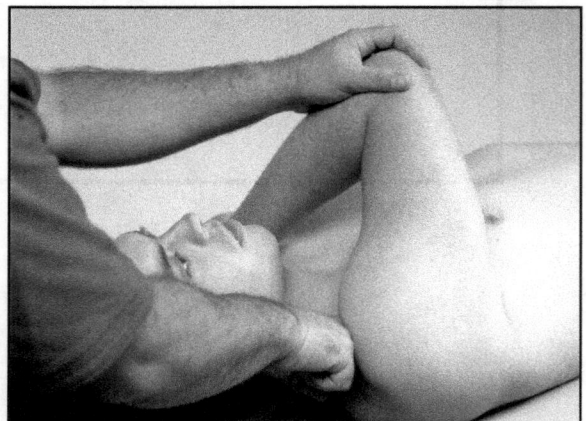

F	████▨▨▨	
Ri	████████	
Ad	████████	

Long Head of Biceps (LHB)

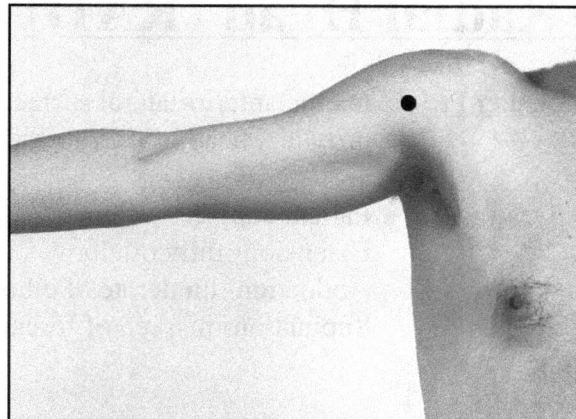

Tender Pt.   5-7 cm lateral to AAC on the tendon of the long head of biceps.

Bursa (BUR)

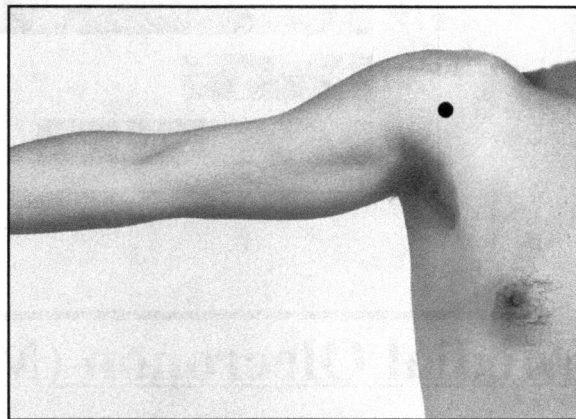

Tender Pt.   3-5 cm lateral to and just below AAC.

Treatment for Long Head of Biceps and Bursa:

Treatment   Patient supine.
Flexion- shoulder 90°, Fully and gently flex elbow
Rotation- internally or externally for comfort

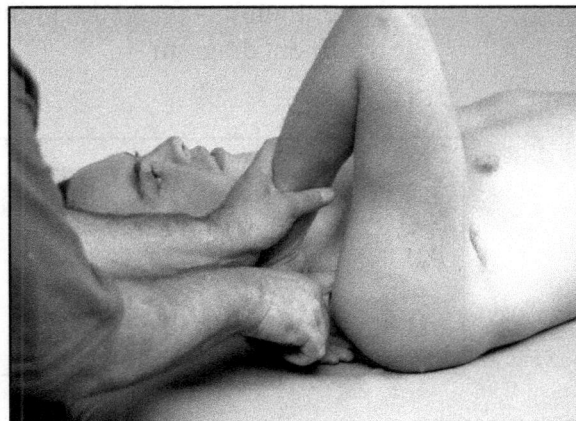

F	▆▆▆▆▆▆▆
Ri/Re	▆▆▆▆

Radial Head (RAD)

Tender Pt.   On the anterio-lateral surface of the proximal head of the radius.

Treatment   Patient supine.
Extension- fully of elbow.
Abduction- moderate of elbow
Supination- marked of forearm

E	████████████
Ab	████████
Su	██████████

Medial Olecronon (MOL)

Tender Pt.   On the medial aspect of the olecronon behind the elbow.

Treatment   Patient supine.
Extension- hyperextension of elbow
Abduction- slight of elbow.
Supination- moderate

Note: thumb is on tender point in treatment diagram

E	██████████████
Ab	████
Su	██████

56

Lateral Olecronon (LOL)

Tender Pt.   On the lateral aspect of the olecronon behind the elbow.

Treatment   Patient supine.
Extension- hyperextension of elbow
Adduction- slight of elbow.
Supination- moderate

Note: Middle finger is on tender point in treatment diagram

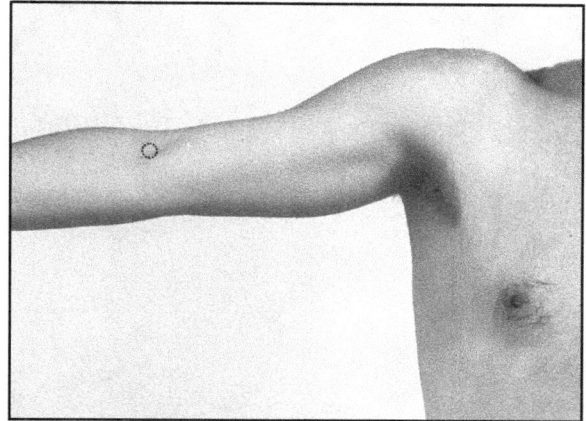

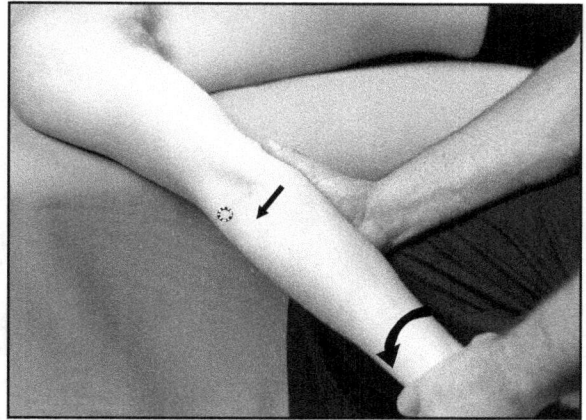

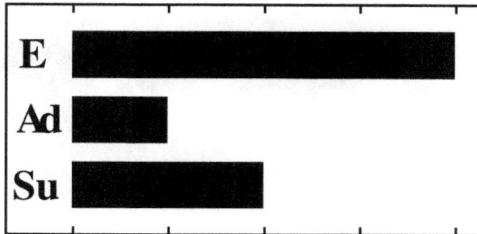

E	████████████████
Ad	███
Su	██████

Lateral and Medial Coronoid (LCND & MCND)

Tender Pts.   Lateral and medial surface of coronoid process.

Treatment   Patient Supine.
Flexion- marked of elbow and shoulder
Rotation- external of humerus
Pronation- marked of radius

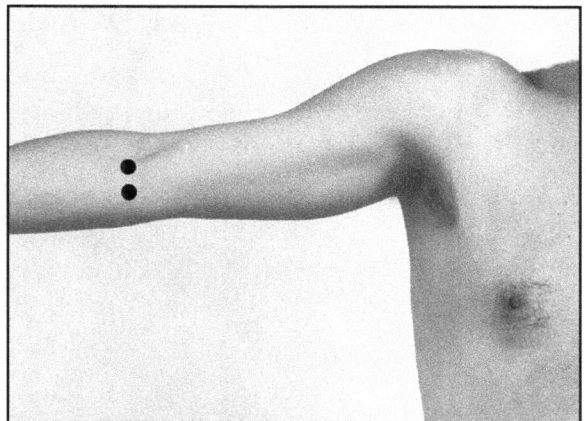

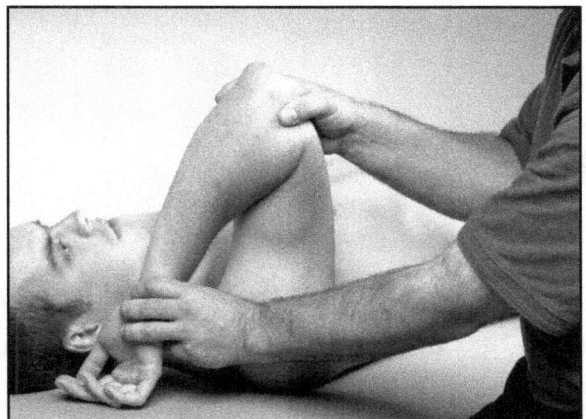

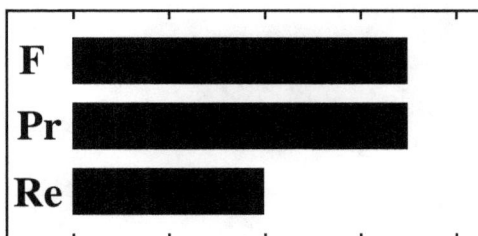

F	███████████████
Pr	███████████████
Re	███████

<u>Notes</u>

Wrist and Hand
Tender Points

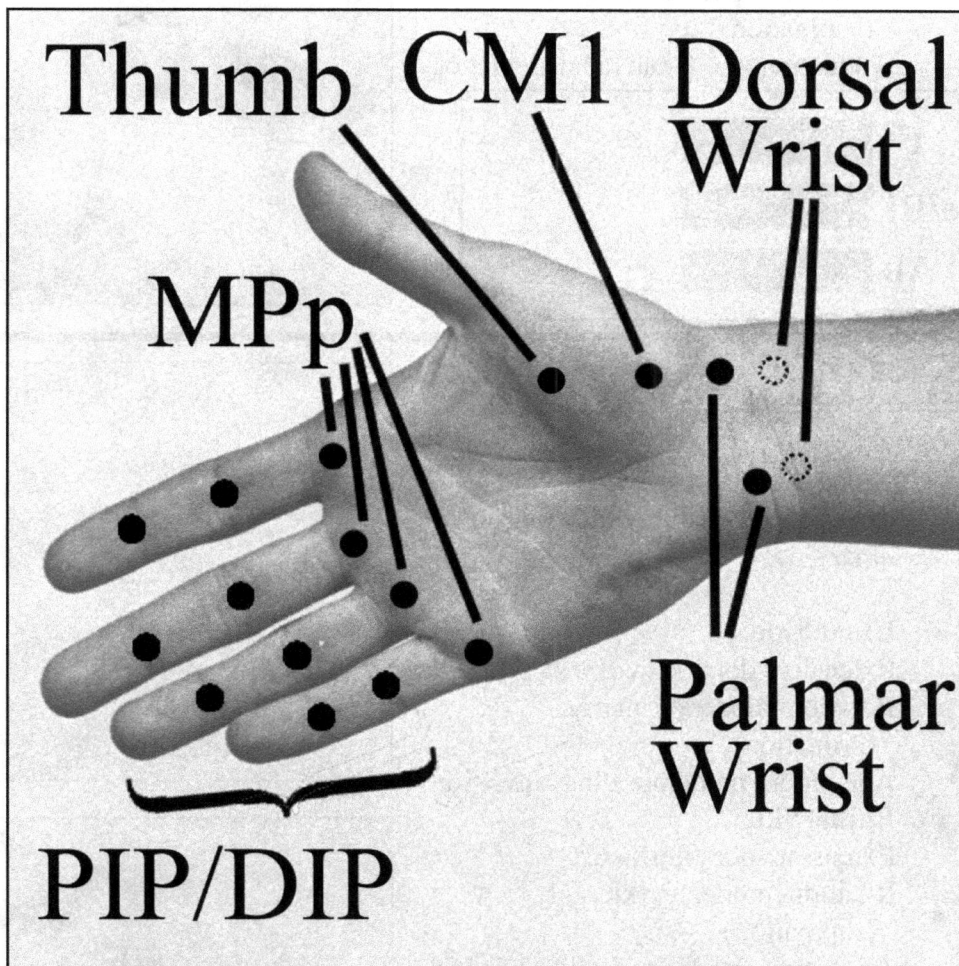

Thumb CM1 Dorsal Wrist

MPp

PIP/DIP

Palmar Wrist

Palmar Wrist (PW)

Tender Pts.   On or just distal to the palmar wrist creases on either the radial or ulnar side.

Treatment   **Ulnar Side:**
Flexion- palmarflex wrist
Rotation- moderate internal (pronation)
Adduction- moderate ulnar deviation
Radial Side:
Flexion- palmarflex wrist
Rotation- moderate external (supination)
Abduction- moderate radial deviation

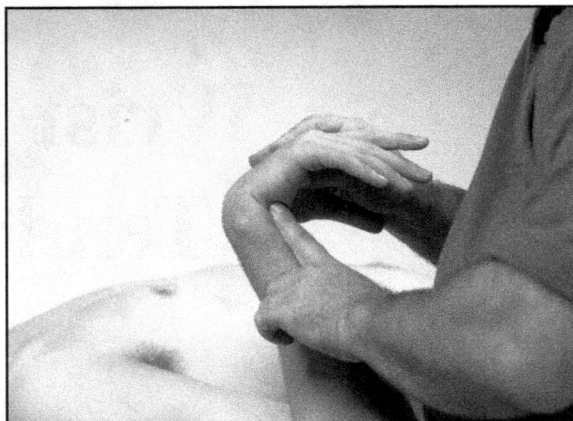

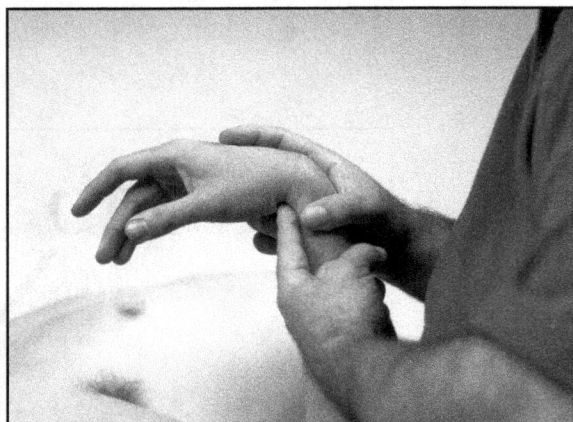

F	■■■■
Re/Ri	■■■■
Ad/Ab	■■■■

Dorsal Wrist (DW)

Tender Pts.   Along dorsal wrist creases of the carpal bones on either the radial or ulnar side.

Treatment   **Ulnar Side:**
Extension- dorsiflex wrist
Rotation- moderate internal (pronation)
Adduction- moderate ulnar deviation
Radial Side:
Extension- dorsiflex wrist
Rotation- moderate external (supination)
Abduction- moderate radial deviation

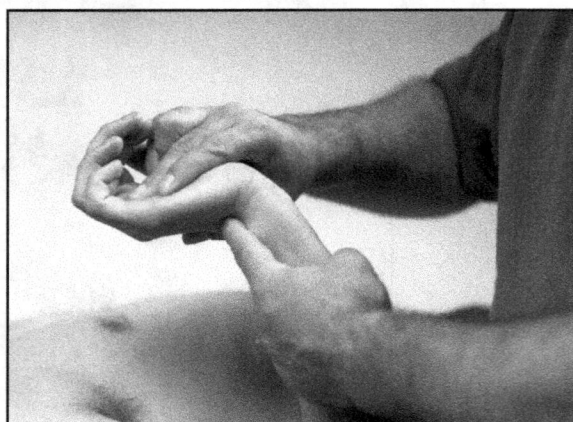

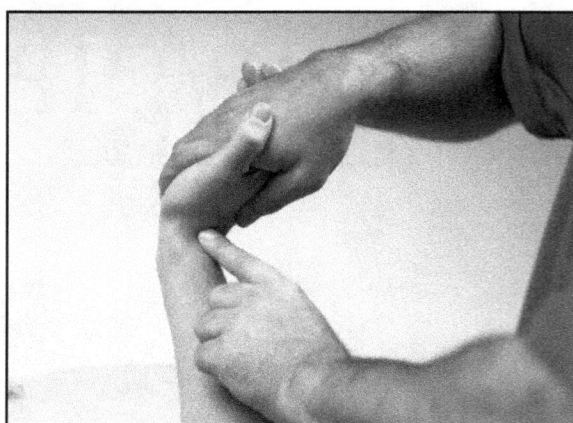

E	■■■■
Re/Ri	■■■■
Ad/Ab	■■■■

Tender Point Locations for Palmar and Dorsal Wrist

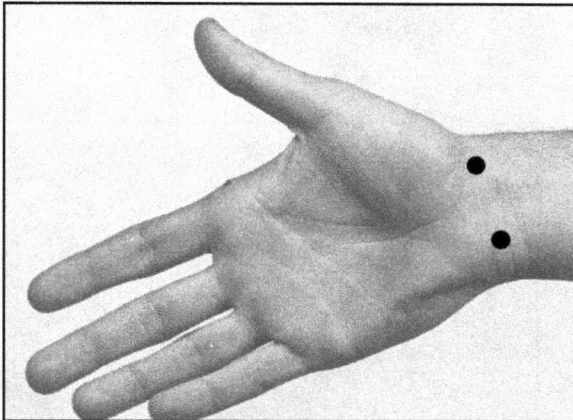

Palmar Points

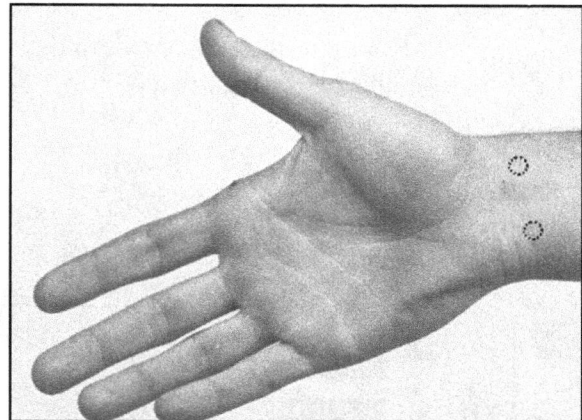

**Dorsal Points
(posterior)**

First Carpometacarpal (CM1)

Tender Pt.   In the palm at the proximal end of the first metacarpal.

Treatment   Flexion- marked palmar flexion of wrist
              Adduction- moderate of the thumb

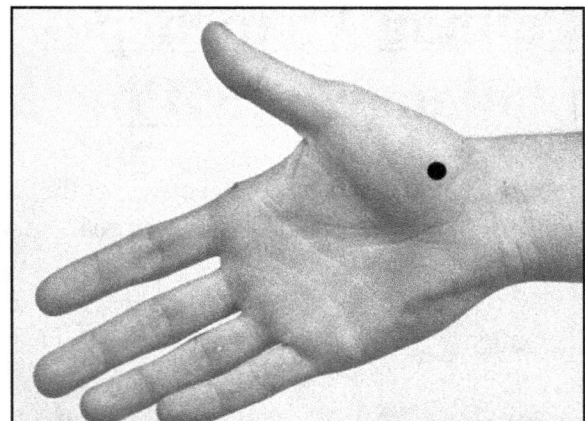

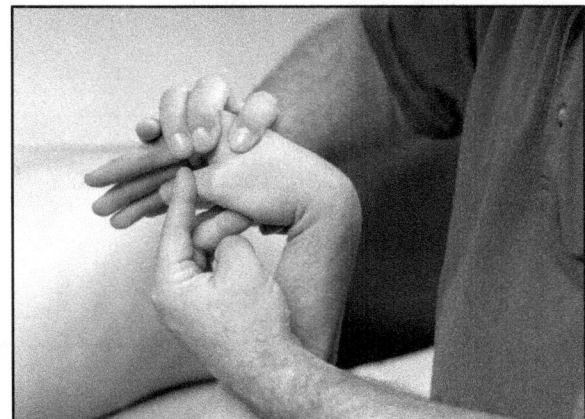

F	████████████
Ad	███████

Thumb

Tender Pt. In the medial adductor muscle mass of the thumb.

Treatment Approximate the thumb to the palm.
Flexion- moderate of the metacarpal phalangeal joint
Rotation- internal or external of thumb for maximal comfort

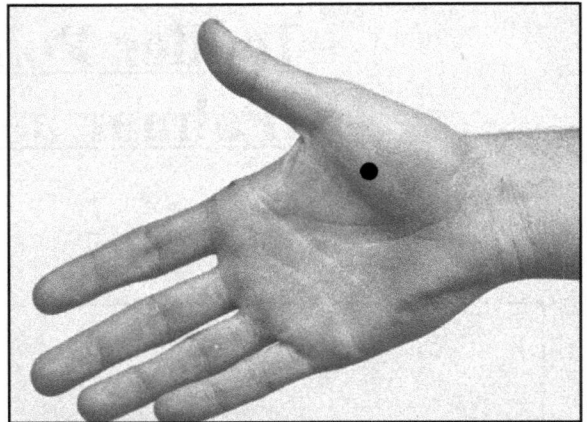

F				
Ri/Re				

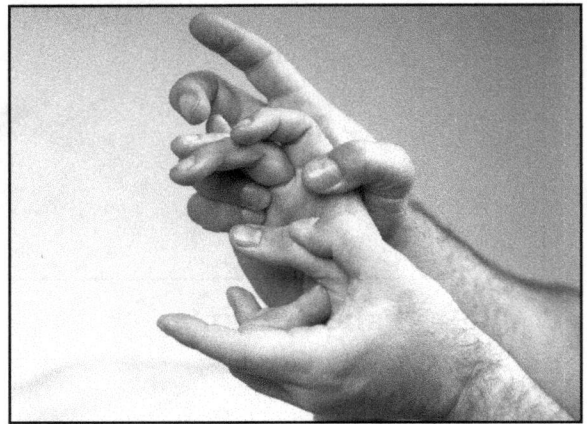

Palmar Metacarpo-phalangeal (MPp)

Tender Pt. On the palmar surface of the shafts of the phalangeal bones near the MP joints.

Treatment Flexion- marked at MP joint
Sidebend- toward
Rotate- internal or external for maximal relief

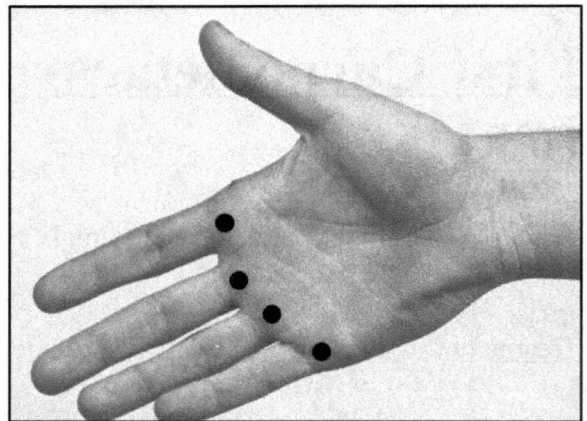

F				
St				
Re/Ri				

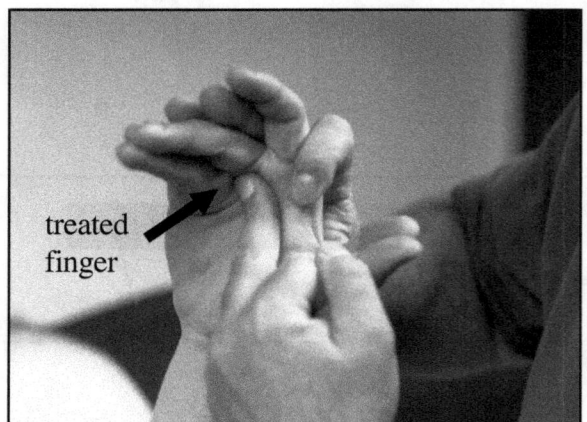

treated finger

Palmar Interphalangeal (PIP) or Flexed Interphalangeal (FIP)

Tender Pt.   On the palmar surface of the shafts of the phalangeal bones near the IP joints.

Treatment   Flexion- marked at IP joint
Sidebend- toward
Rotate- internal or external for maximal relief

F	████████████
St	████████
Re/Ri	████

Dorsal Interphalangeal (DIP) or Extension Interphalangeal (EIP)

Tender Pt.   On the dorsal surface of the shafts of the phalangeal bones near the IP joints.

Treatment   Extension- moderate to marked at IP joint
Sidebend- toward
Rotate- internal or external for maximal relief

E	██████████░░░░
St	█████████
Re/Ri	████

63

Notes

Tender Points of the Hip

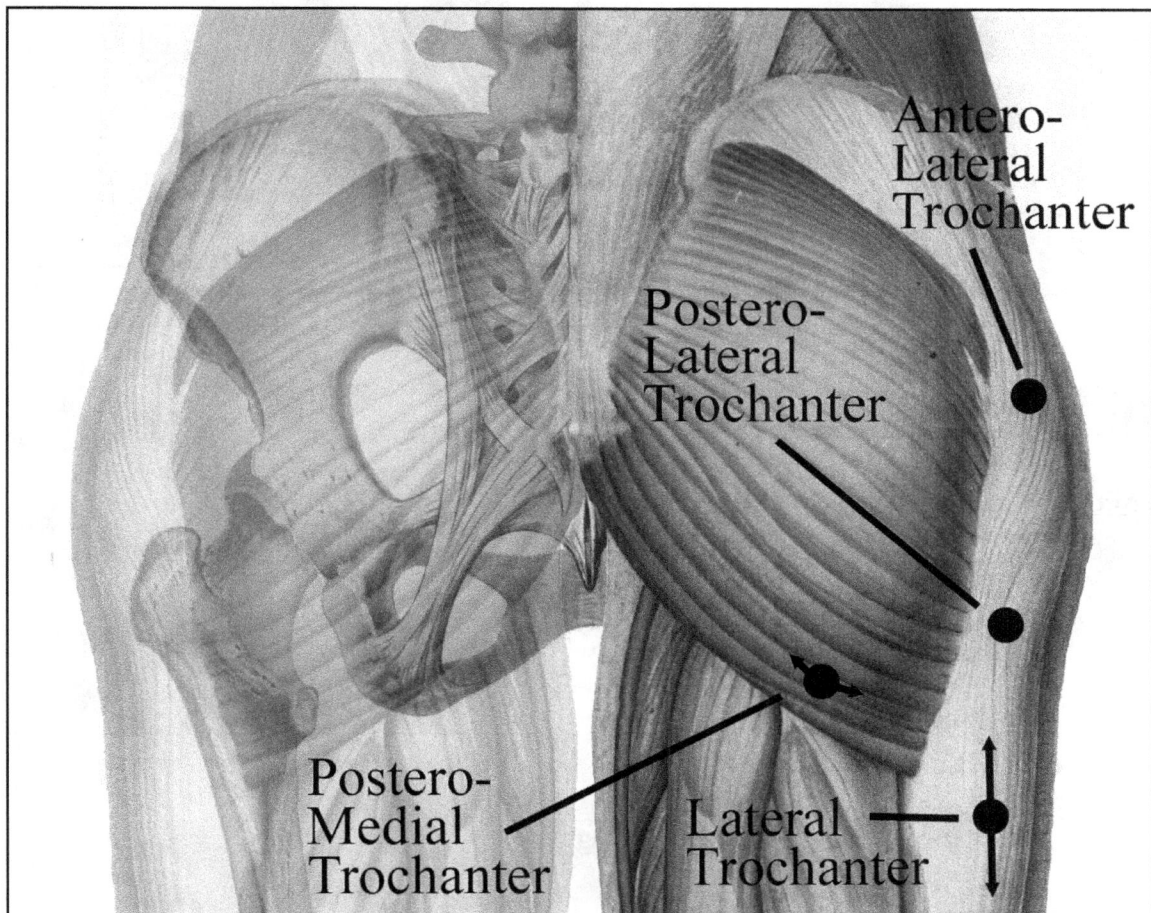

Antero-
Lateral
Trochanter

Postero-
Lateral
Trochanter

Postero-
Medial
Trochanter

Lateral
Trochanter

Lateral Trochanter (LT)

Tender Pt. On the lateral surface of the femur, 0-15 cm. distal from the greater trochanter along a line in the iliotibial band.

Treatment Patient prone. Operator seated supporting patient's leg on his thigh.
Flexion- slight of the hip
Abduction- moderate of thigh
Rotation- may need internal rotation

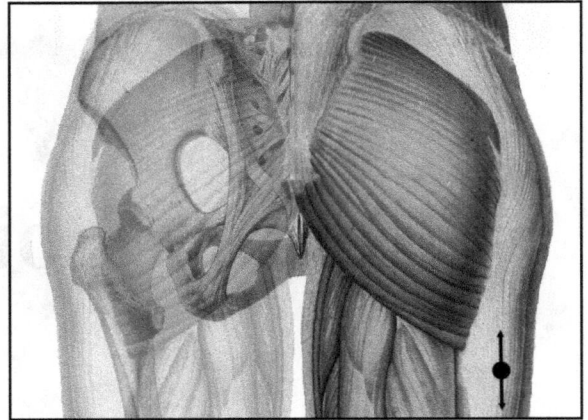

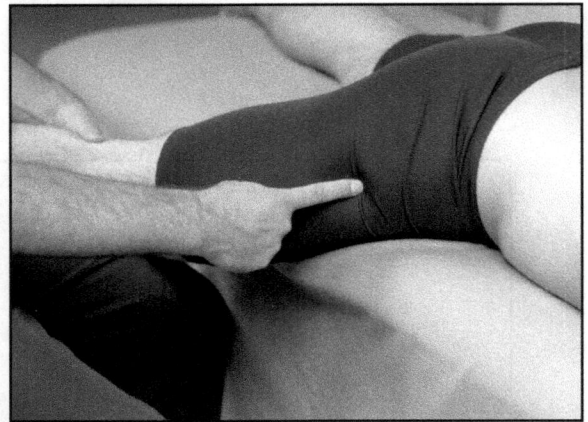

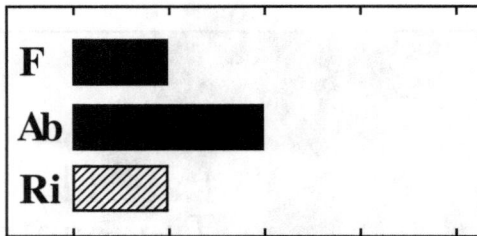

Postero-Lateral Trochanter (PLT)

Tender Pt. On the superior-lateral aspect of the posterior surface of the greater trochanter.

Treatment Patient prone. Operator standing with knee on table under the lateral aspect of patient's thigh.
Extension- moderate of the hip
Abduction- slight
Rotation- marked externally of thigh

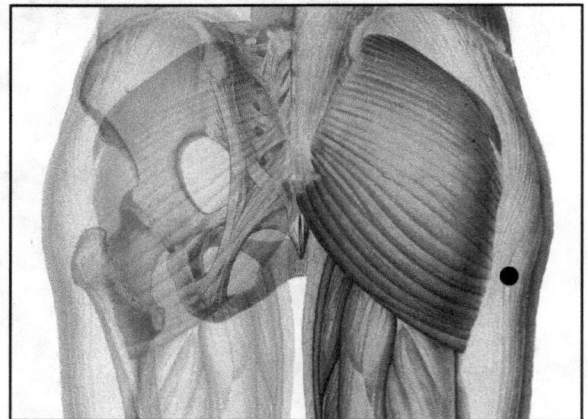

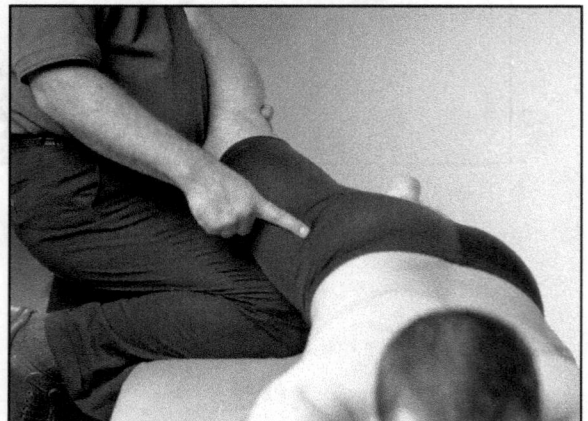

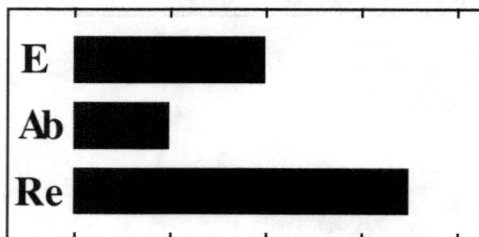

Postero-Medial Trochanter (PMT)

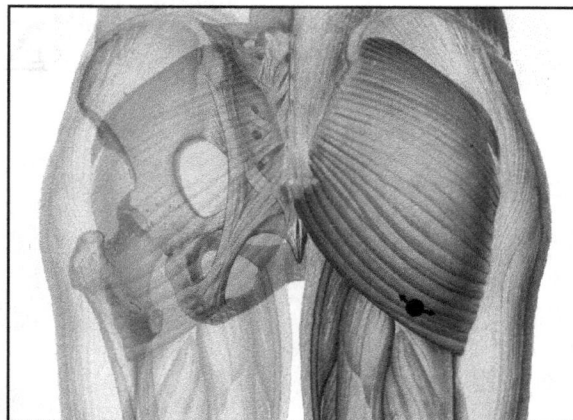

Tender Pt.   3-5 mm inferior to the trochanter between the posterior medial surface of the femur shaft and the posterior lateral surface of the ischial tuberosity.

Treatment   Patient prone. Operator grasps patient's leg standing on same side as dysfunction placing knee under patient's thigh.
Extension- slight
Rotation- moderate externally of thigh
Adduction- usually slight of hip by pulling leg across midline.

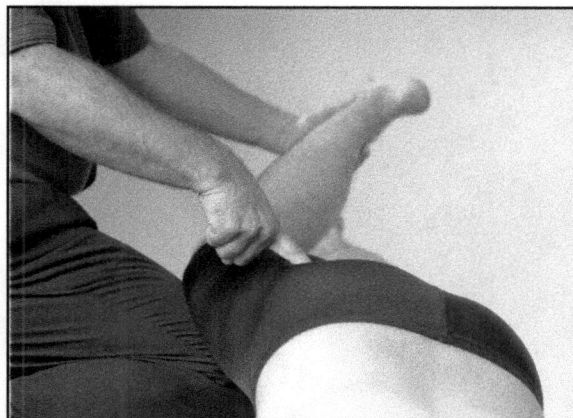

E	████
Re	██████
Ad	███

Antero-Lateral Trochanter (ALT)

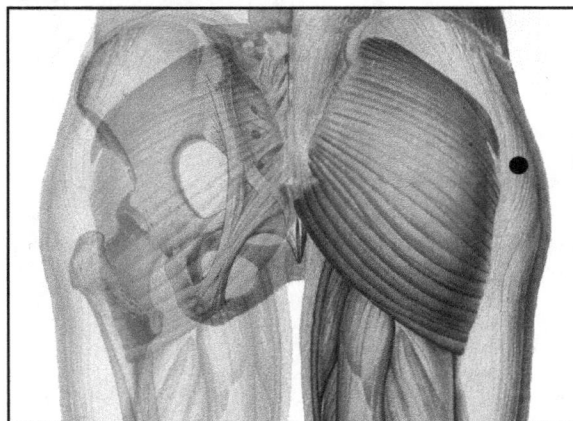

Tender Pt.   5-7 cm. lateral and inferior to the ASIS, anterior and superior to the greater trochanter.

Treatment   Patient supine.
Flexion- of the hip 70-90°
Abduction- moderate of the thigh
Rotation- slight externally of thigh

F	█████
Ab	█████
Re	███

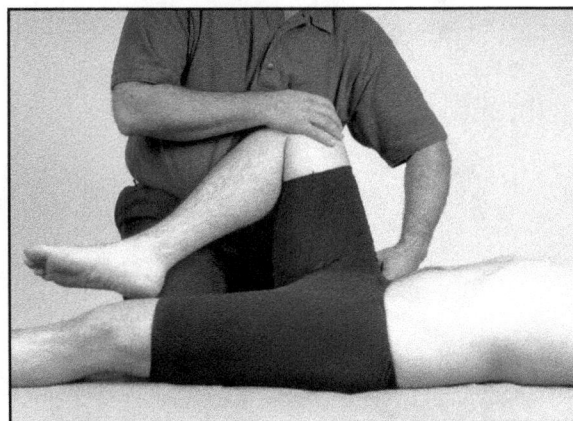

Notes

Anterior Knee Tender Points

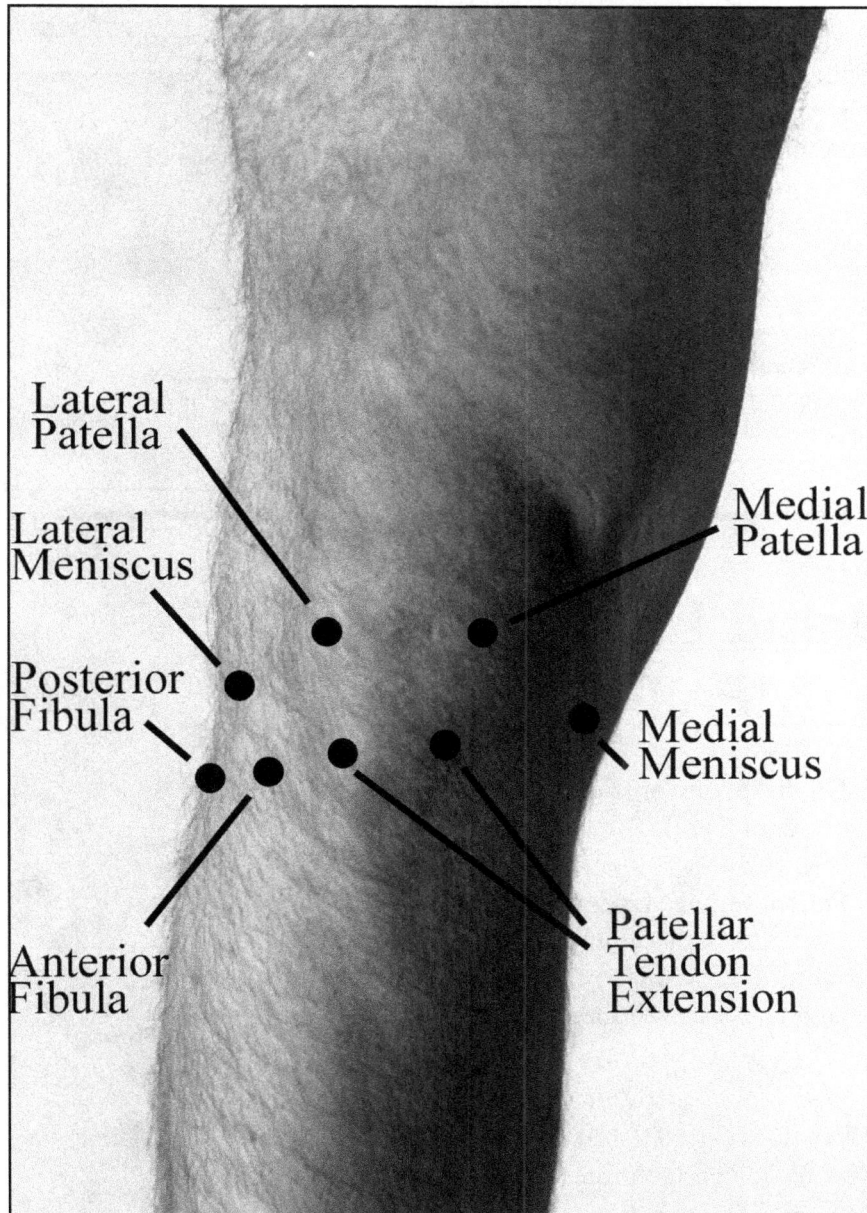

Lateral
Patella

Lateral
Meniscus

Posterior
Fibula

Anterior
Fibula

Medial
Patella

Medial
Meniscus

Patellar
Tendon
Extension

Patellar Tendon Extension (PTE)

Tender Pt.   On the lateral or medial side of the patellar tendon inferior to the patella.

Treatment   Patient supine with leg on table and pillow under ankle. Alternatively, the knee can be extended by lifting leg at ankle.
Extension- hyperextend knee by pressure on the distal femur
Rotation- of the tibia, internal for lateral TP, external for medial TP

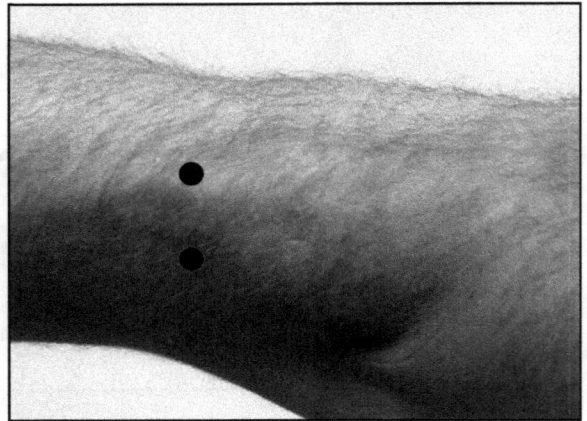

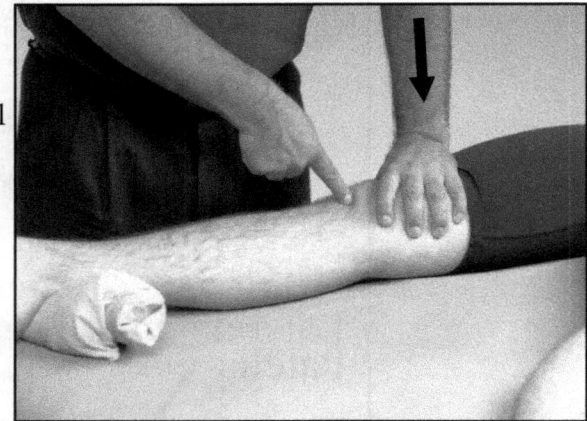

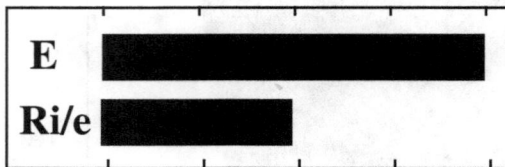

E	████████████████
Ri/e	██████

Medial and Lateral Patella (MPAT & LPAT)

Tender Pts.   On the medial or lateral margin of the center of patella.

Treatment   Patient supine. Operator induces sideward displacement of patella by exerting force on the opposite side of patella towards the tender point.

Note: Leg and foot do not need to be supported with a pillow as in PTE technique.

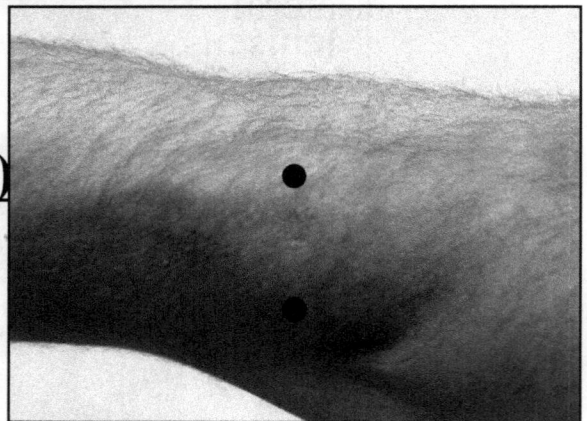

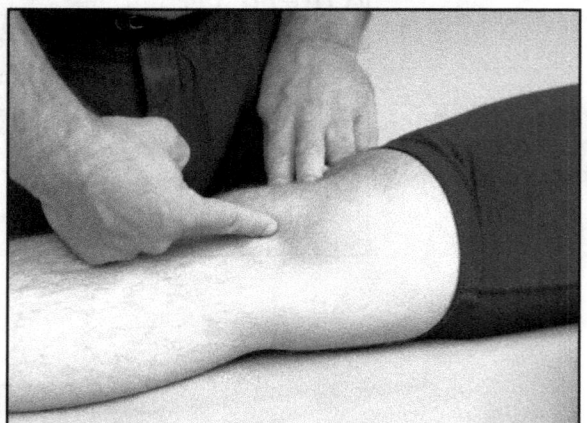

Medial Meniscus (MM)

Tender Pt.   On the medial joint space, usually 5 cm medial and posterior to the medial border of patella.

Treatment   Patient supine with leg off table.
Flexion- knee flexed 40°-80°
Adduction- slight of the tibia
Rotation- moderate internal of the tibia

Note: Ankle plantar flexion and inversion.

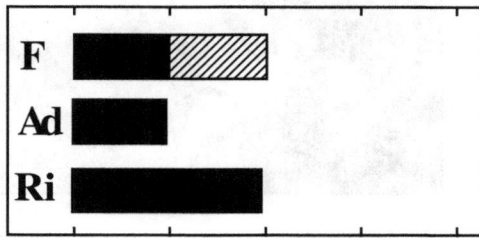

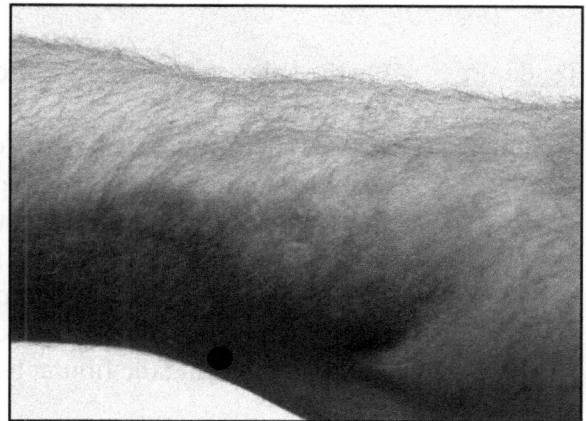

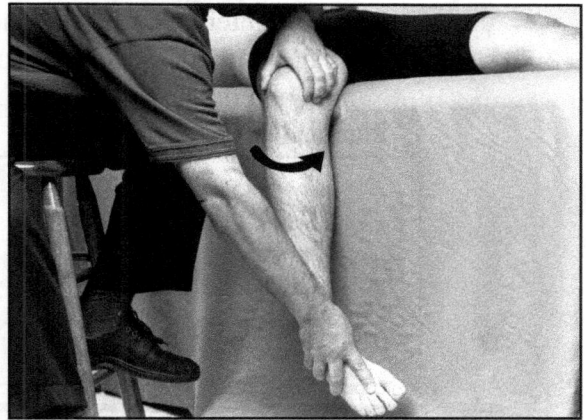

F	███████░░░	
Ad	█████	
Ri	███████	

Lateral Meniscus (LM)

Tender Pt.   On the lateral joint space, usually 5 cm lateral and posterior to the inferior lateral border of patella.

Treatment   Patient supine with leg off table.
Flexion- knee flexed 40°-80°
Abduction- slight of tibia
Rotation-moderate external

Note: Ankle dorsiflexion and eversion.

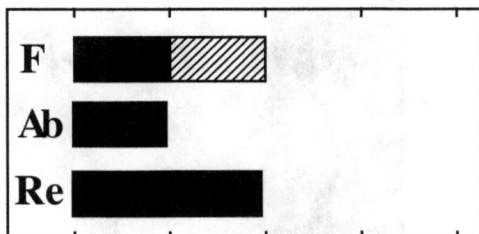

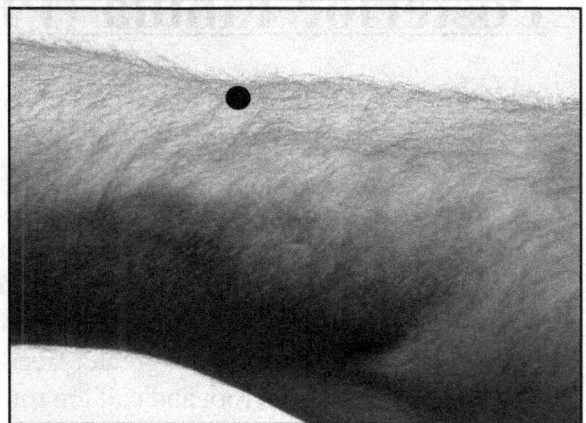

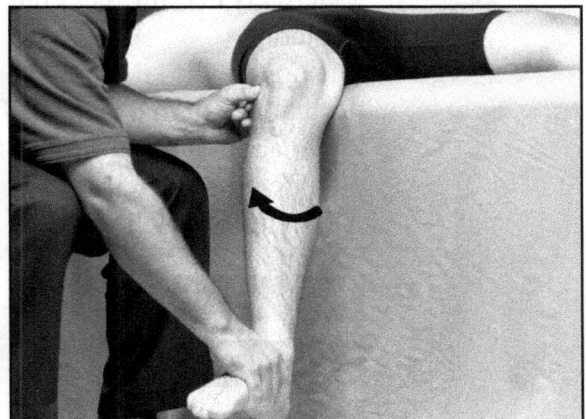

F	██████░░░	
Ab	█████	
Re	████████	

Anterior Fibula (AFIB)

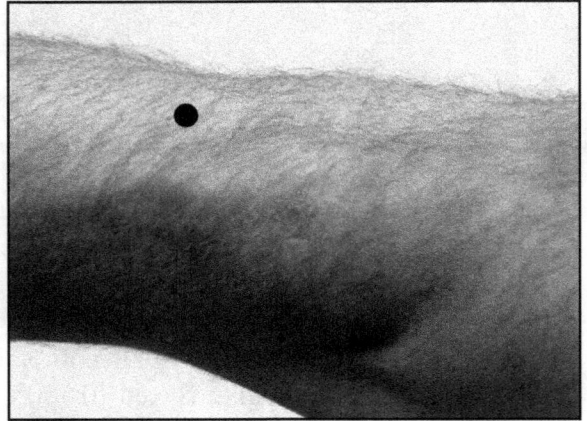

Tender Pt.   On the anterior aspect of the proximal fibular head.

Treatment   Patient supine or seated, operator seated on same side as tender point. Patient's knee bent 80-90°, foot is inverted to "gap" the proximal fibular head to allow it greater freedom of motion, foot and calf are rotated internally to bring the fibular head forward.

Flexion- of the knee 80-90°

Rotation- internal of the calf and foot

Supination- moderate of the foot with ankle inversion.

Plantarflexion- of the ankle

F	████████
Ri	████████
Su	████████

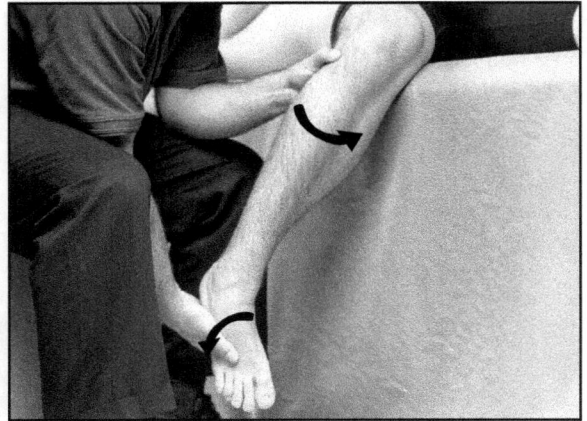

Posterior Fibula (PFIB)

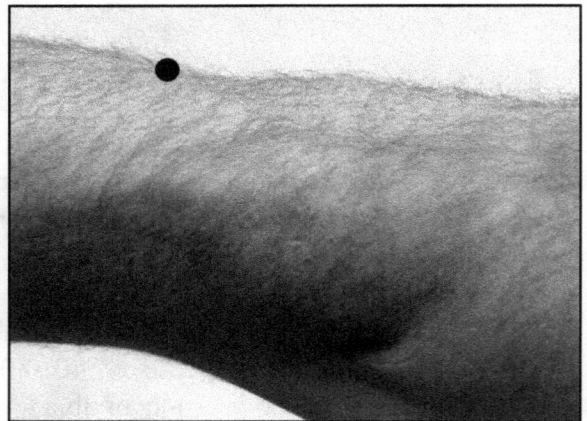

Tender Pt.   On the posterior aspect of the proximal fibular head.

Treatment   Patient supine or seated, operator seated on same side as tender point. Patient's knee bent 80-90°, foot is inverted to "gap" the proximal fibular head to allow it greater freedom of motion, foot and calf are rotated externally to bring the fibular head posterior.

Flexion- of the knee 80-90°

Rotation- external of the calf and foot

Supination- moderate of the foot with ankle inversion.

Dorsiflexion- of the ankle

F	████████
Re	████████
Su	████████

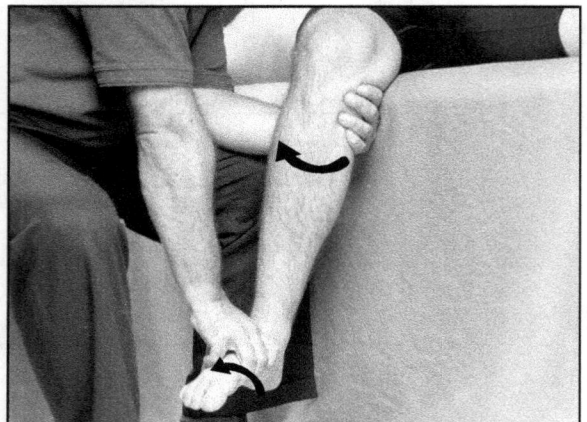

Posterior Knee Tender Points

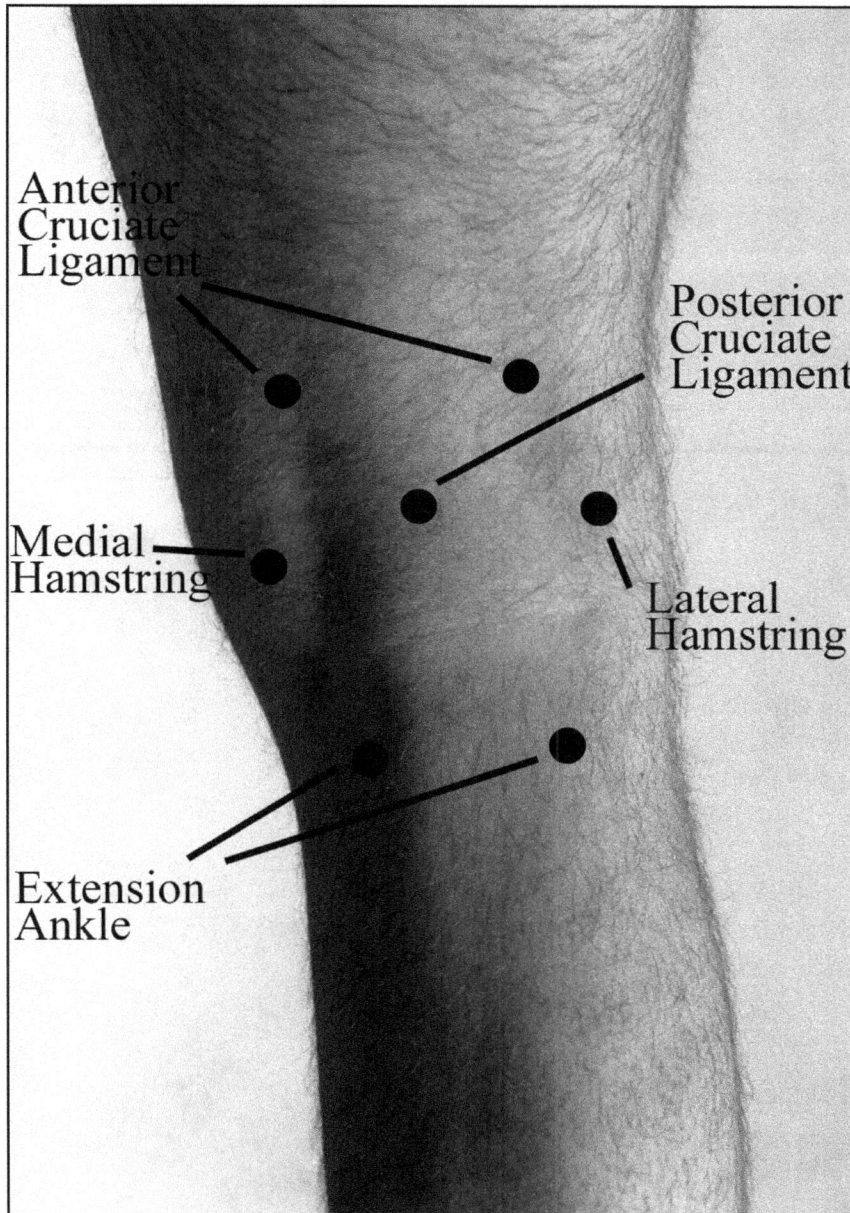

Anterior Cruciate Ligament

Posterior Cruciate Ligament

Medial Hamstring

Lateral Hamstring

Extension Ankle

Medial Hamstring (MH)

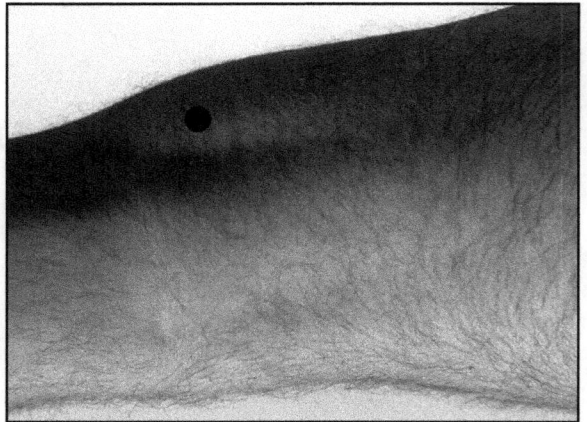

Tender Pt.   On the medial hamstring near the distal attachment.

Treatment   Patient supine. Operator stands on same side as tender point with caudad foot on the table. Patient's foot is held in operator's flexed knee.
Flexion- of knee about 60°
Rotation- moderate externally of tibia by exerting medialward and upward pressure on calcaneus.
Adduction- slight of the calcaneus

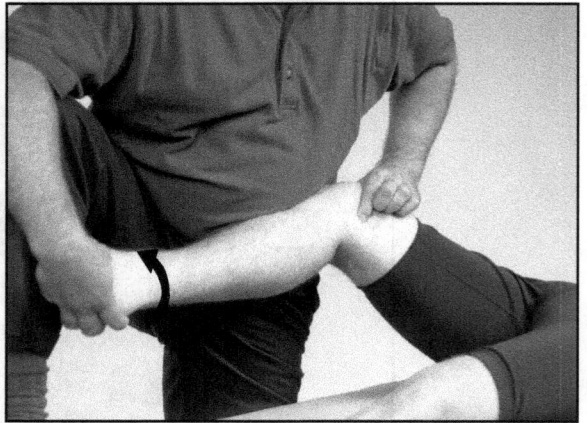

```
F   ████████████
Re  ████████████
Ad  █████
```

Lateral Hamstring (LH)

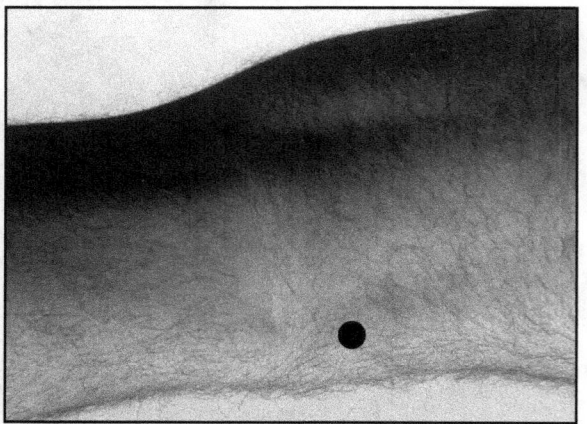

Tender Pt.   On the lateral hamstring at the distal attachment near the fibular head.

Treatment   Patient supine with leg off the table.
Flexion- slight of knee about 30°
Rotation- moderate externally
Abduction- slight of the tibia

Note: Same as lateral meniscus treatment with less flexion and more external rotation.

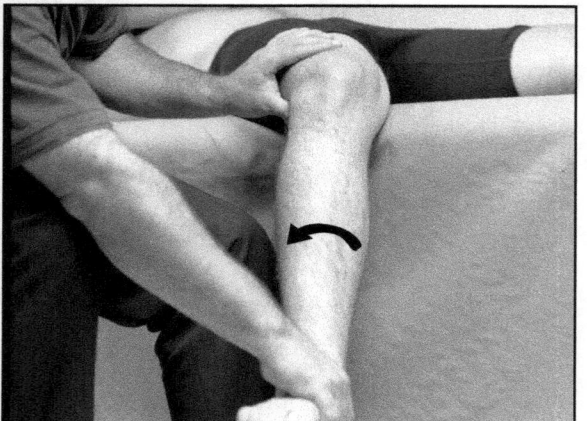

```
F   ██████
Re  ████████████
Ab  ██████
```

Anterior Cruciate Ligament (ACL)

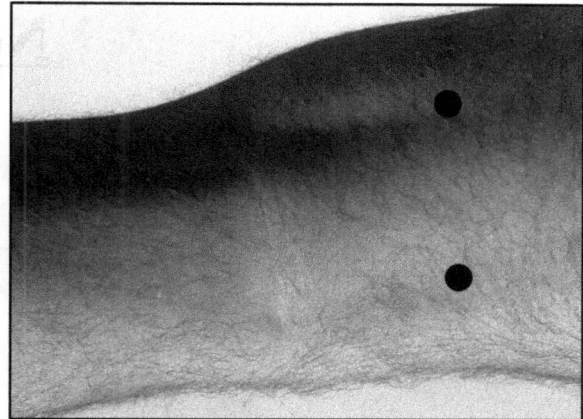

Tender Pt. On either the medial or lateral hamstring in the superior popliteal area.

Treatment Patient supine with pillow under <u>femur</u>. Operator stands on same side as tender point and places downward pressure on anterior tibia immediately below knee.
Extension- moderate of the knee
Rotation- slight internal of tibia
Adduction- sometimes slight of tibia

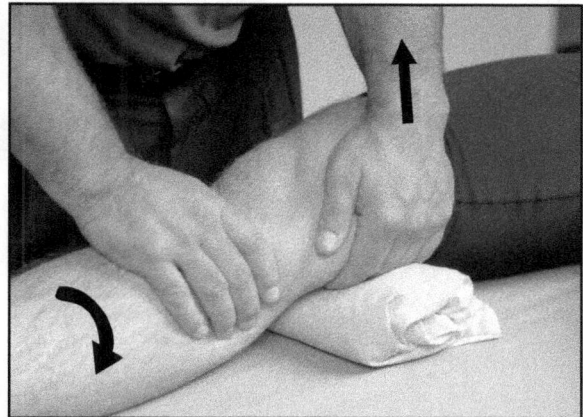

E	
Ri	
Ad	

Posterior Cruciate Ligament (PCL)

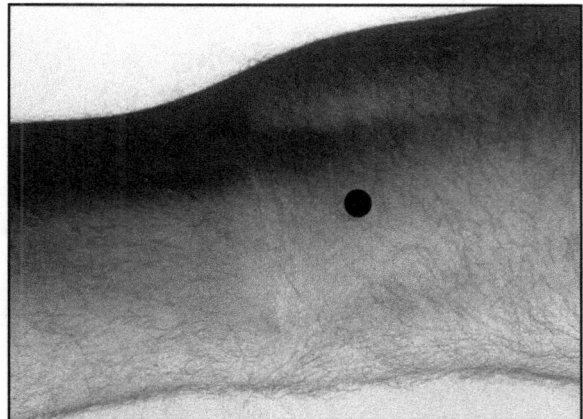

Tender Pt. In the middle of the popliteal space.

Treatment Patient supine with pillow under <u>tibia</u>. Operator stands on same side as tender point and places downward pressure on anterior femur immediately above knee.
Extension- moderate of the knee
Rotation- slight internal of tibia
Adduction- sometimes slight of femur

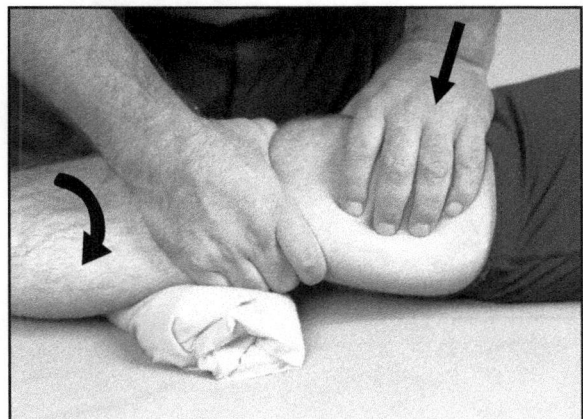

E	
Ri	
Ad	

<u>Notes</u>

Tender Points of the Foot and Ankle

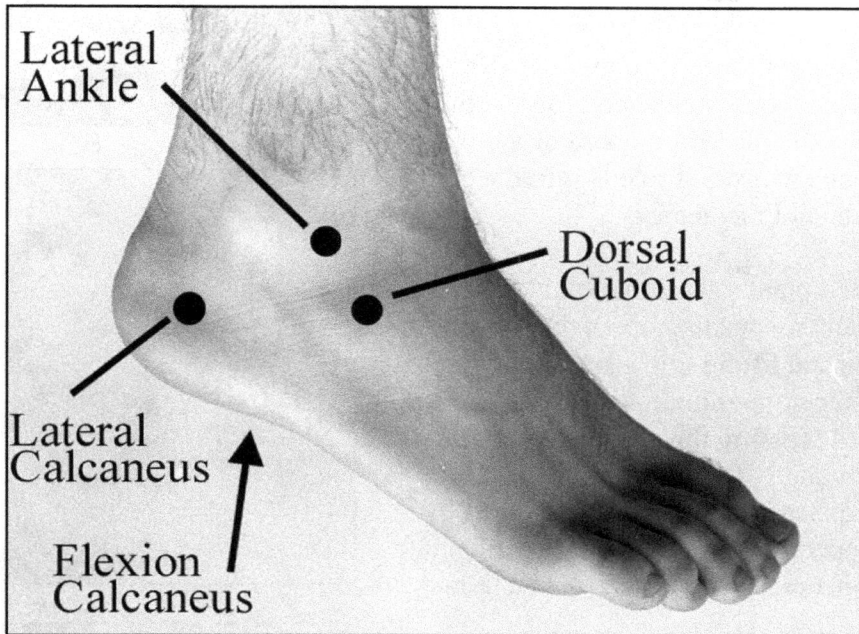

Lateral Ankle
Dorsal Cuboid
Lateral Calcaneus
Flexion Calcaneus

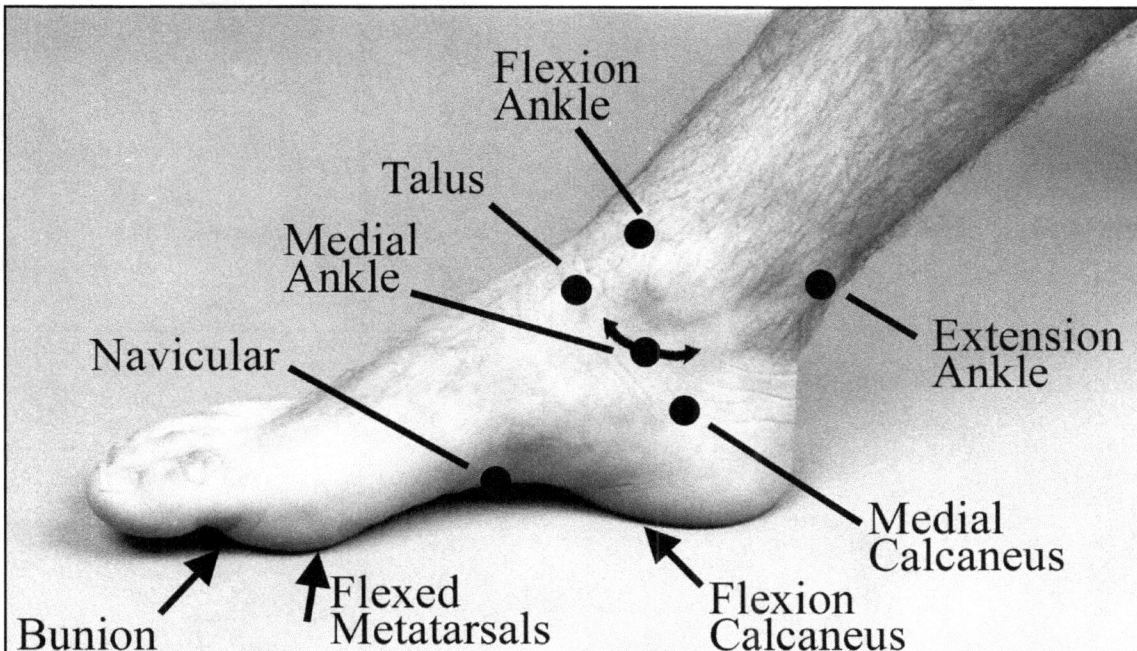

Flexion Ankle
Talus
Medial Ankle
Navicular
Extension Ankle
Bunion
Flexed Metatarsals
Flexion Calcaneus
Medial Calcaneus

Extension Ankle (EA)

<u>Tender Pts.</u>   1) On the lower margin of the popliteal space on the medial or lateral gastrocnemius
2) On the distal Achilles tendon medially or laterally, usually 3 cm above calcaneus.

<u>Treatment</u>   Patient prone. Operator standing on same side as dysfunction with caudad foot on the table. Patient's foot is placed on operator's proximal thigh near groin so extension force is introduced into the patient's ankle, not metatarsals.

Extension- marked plantar flexion of ankle (not metatarsals) by pushing down on posterior calcaneus and lifting thigh for maximal plantar flexion. Operator simultaneously exerts strong downward pressure through patient's calf with the other hand.

Rotation- slight internal of ankle accomplished by moving operator's knee cephalad while main taining operator's pelvis and foot stationary.

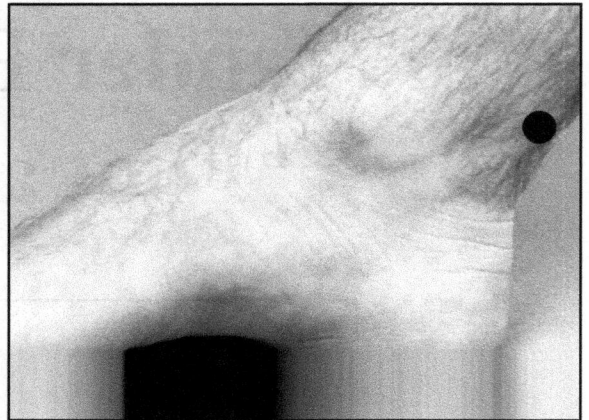

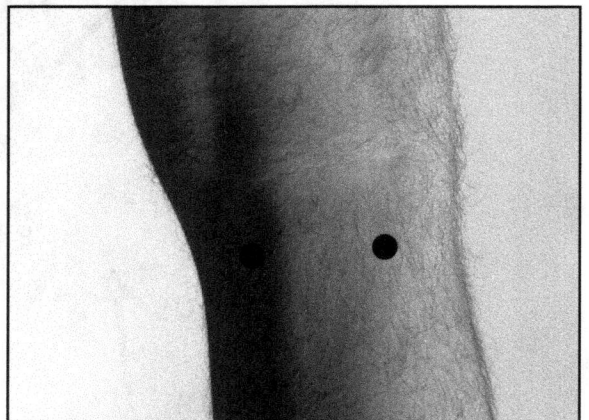

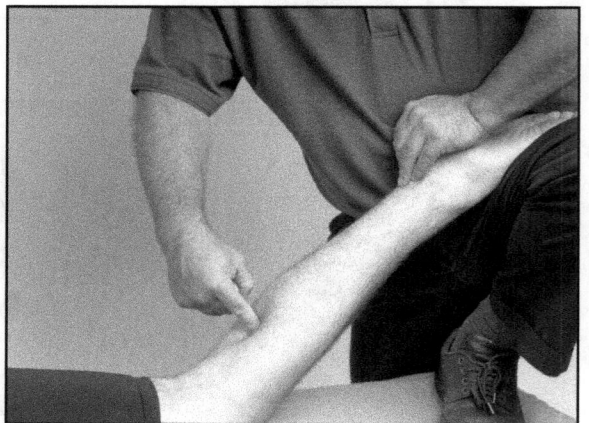

Flexion Ankle (FA)

Tender Pt.   Anterior to the medial malleolus,
              medial to the tendon of the extensor
              digitorum longus.

Treatment   Patient prone with knee flexed about
              90°.
              Flexion- marked dorsiflexion of the
                 ankle

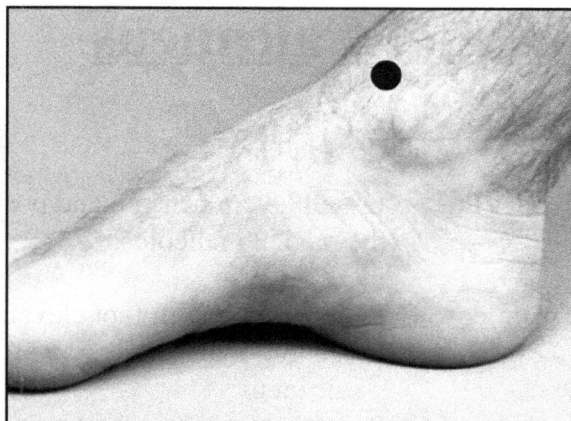

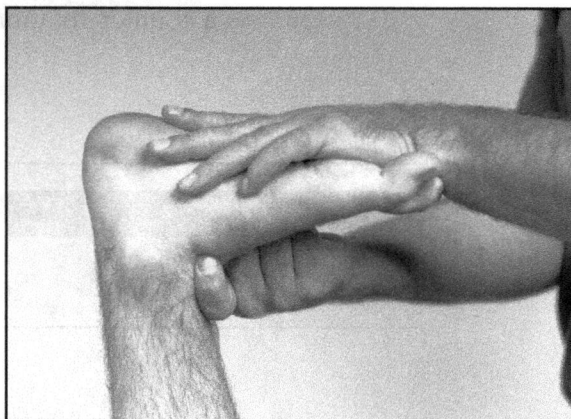

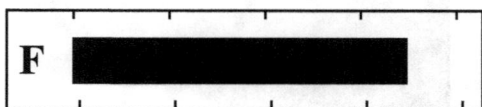

F ████████████████

Medial Ankle (MA)

Tender Pt.   Usually 2 cm beneath the medial
              malleolus in an arc about 2 cm long.

Treatment   Patient prone with foot elevated.
              Inversion- maximal inversion of
                 calcaneus

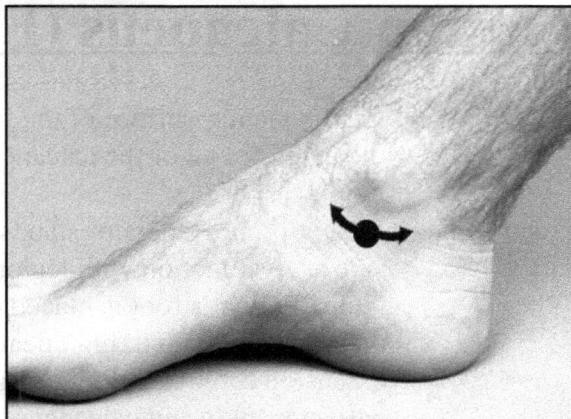

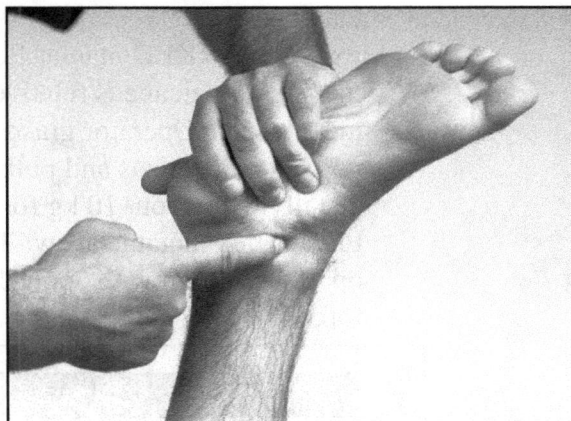

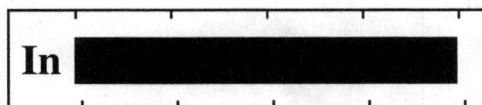

In ████████████████

Medial Calcaneus (MCA)

Tender Pt.   Usually 3 cm beneath and posterior to the medial malleolus.

Treatment   Patient prone with foot elevated.
Inversion- hyper-inversion of calcaneus
Pronation- moderate pronation of forefoot as a counter-rotation

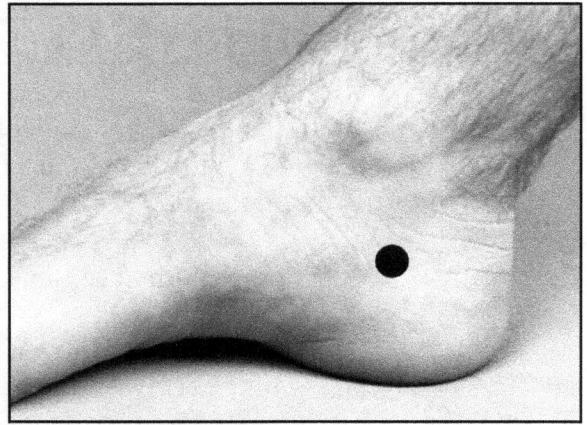

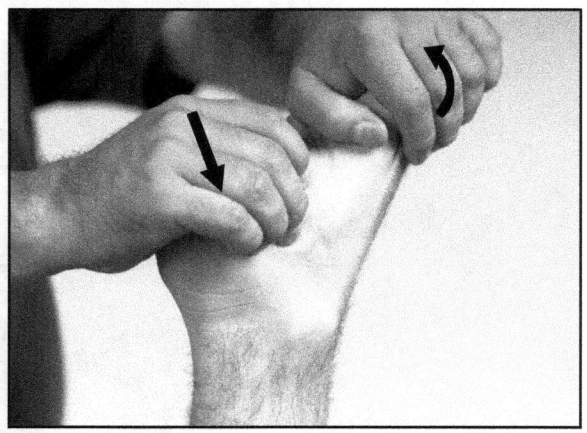

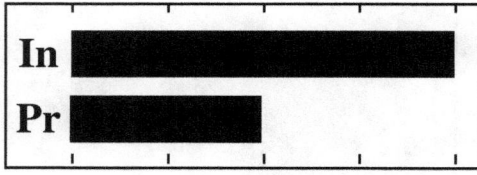

In	
Pr	

Flexion Calcaneus (FCA)

Tender Pt.   On the plantar surface of the foot at the anterior end of the calcaneus.

Treatment   Patient prone. Operator stands on same side as dysfunction with leg on the table. Patient's foot is placed on operator's proximal thigh near groin so extension force is introduced into the patient's ankle and calcaneus, not metatarsals.
Flexion- MARKED plantar flexion of the plantar calcaneus relative to the metatarsals. Operator grasps patient's posterior calcaneus and pulls heel distally with about 10 kg force. Plantar flex metatarsals while lifting operator's thigh with about 15 kg force.

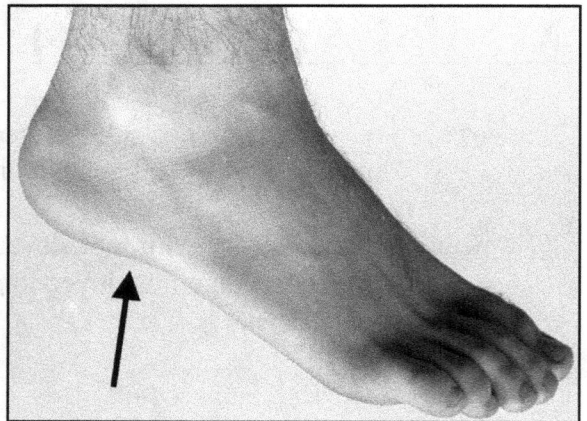

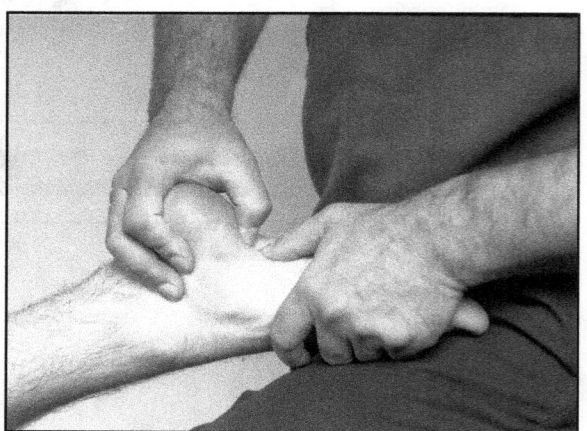

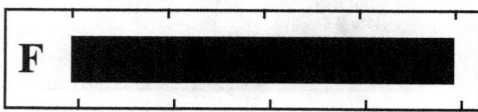

F	

Talus (TAL)

Tender Pt.   On the medial ankle, anterior to the
               medial malleolus on the anterior tip
               of the talus.

Treatment   Patient prone with foot elevated.
               Supination- slight of foot
               Inversion- marked of ankle

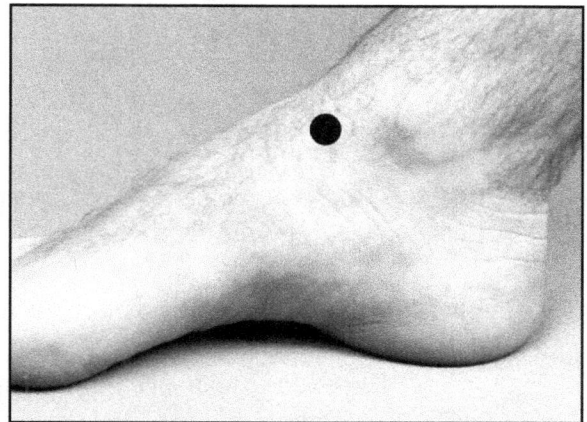

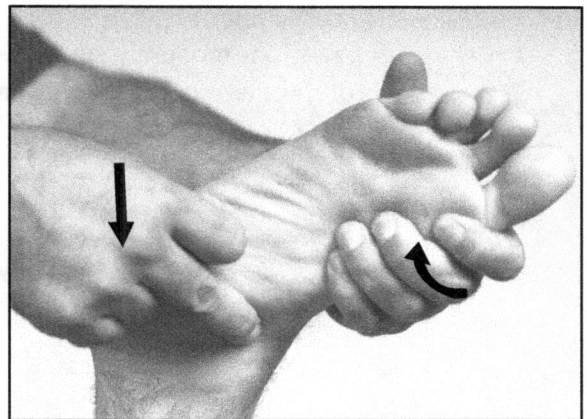

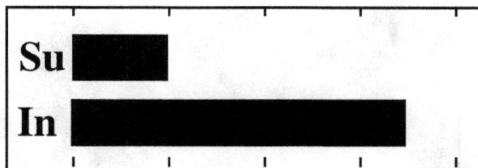

Su					
In					

Lateral Ankle (LA)

Tender Pts.   In a depression, 2 cm anterior and
               inferior to the lateral malleolus.

Treatment   Patient prone with foot elevated.
               Eversion- marked of calcaneus
               Supination- variable

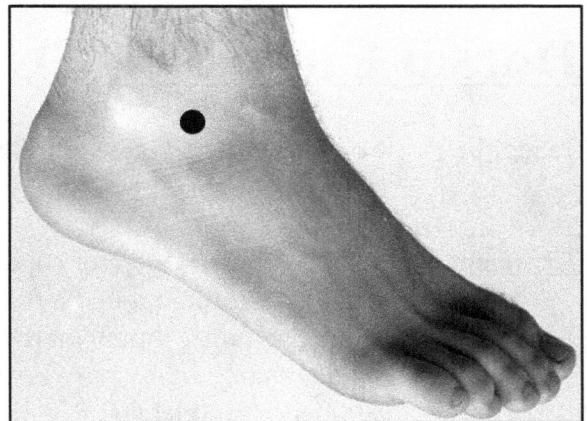

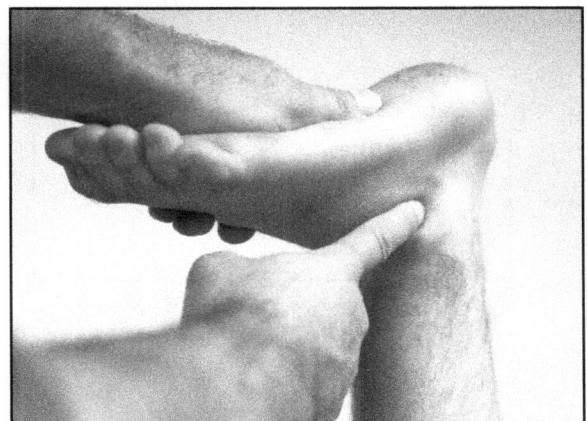

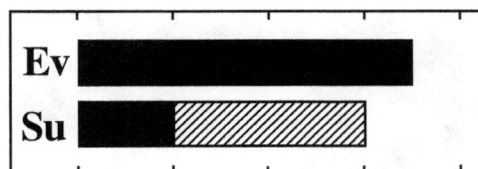

Ev				
Su				

Lateral Calcaneus (LCA)

Tender Pt.   Usually 3 cm beneath and posterior to the lateral malleolus.

Treatment   Patient in supine position with knee extended.
Eversion- hyper-eversion of calcaneus with thumb on medial calcaneus pushing laterally.
Supination- moderate supination of forefoot as a counter rotation.

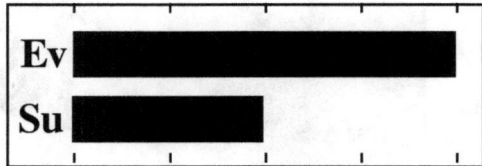

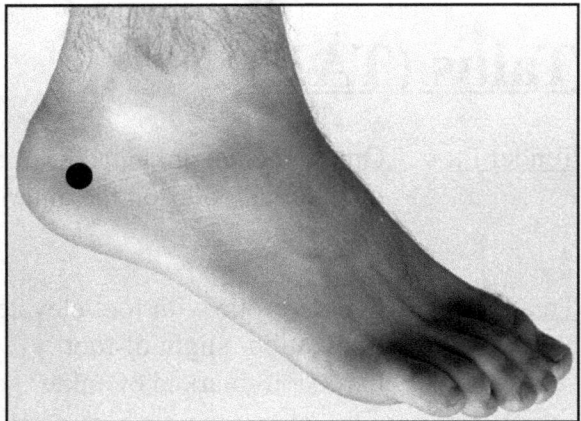

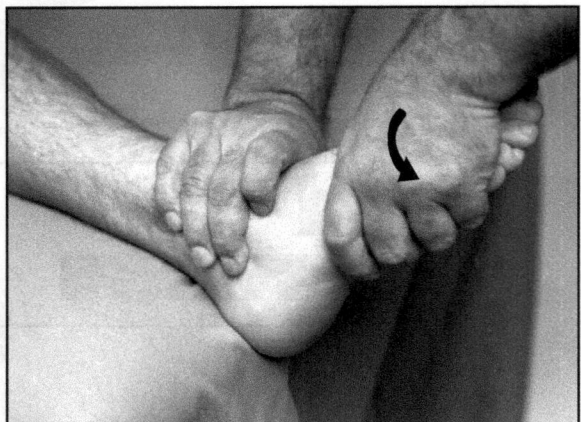

Ev
Su

Dorsal Cuboid (DCU)

Tender Pt.   4 cm anterior and inferior to the lateral malleolus.

Treatment   Patient supine. Operator supinates patient's forefoot around a fulcrum of the operator's thumb on the plantar arch.
Supination- moderate of forefoot
Inversion- moderate of ankle

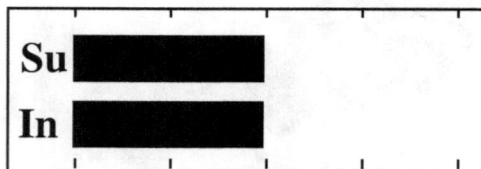

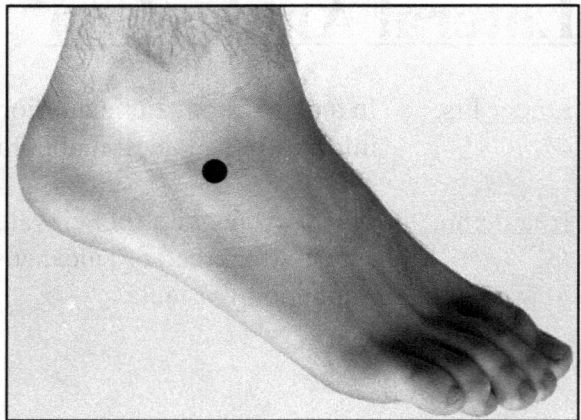

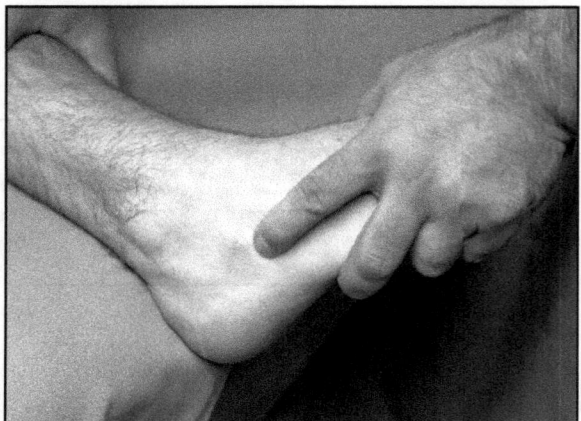

Su
In

Navicular (NAV)

Tender Pt.   Plantar surface of the foot near the apex of the medial arch on the medial or plantar surface of the navicular.

Treatment   Patient prone with foot elevated. Doctor wraps foot around tender point.
Flexion- usually plantar, around the navicular
Supination- of the forefoot
Inversion- moderate of ankle

F	
Su	
In	

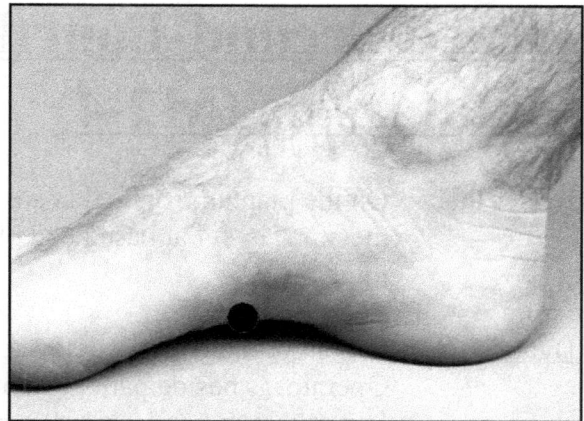

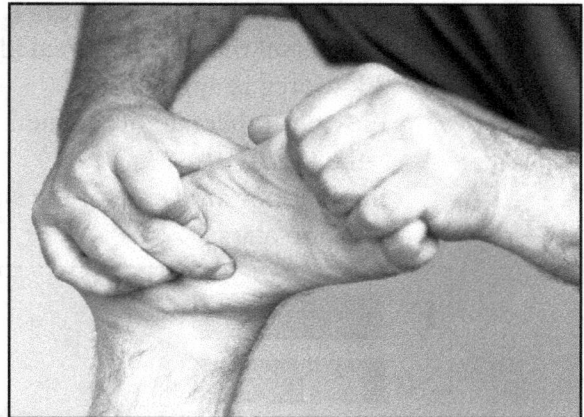

Flexed First Metatarsal (M1)

Tender Pt.   On the lateral shaft of the first metatarsal, proximal to the MT joint.

Treatment   Patient prone with foot elevated. Doctor is beside patient stabilizing foot with one hand and supinating the great toe and first metatarsal.
Supination- of the great toe and first metatarsal with about 3 kg force

| Su | |

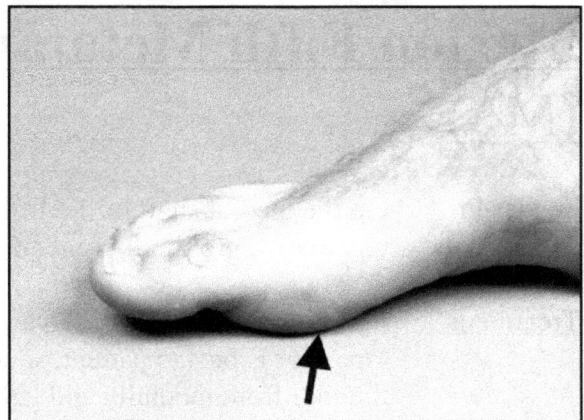

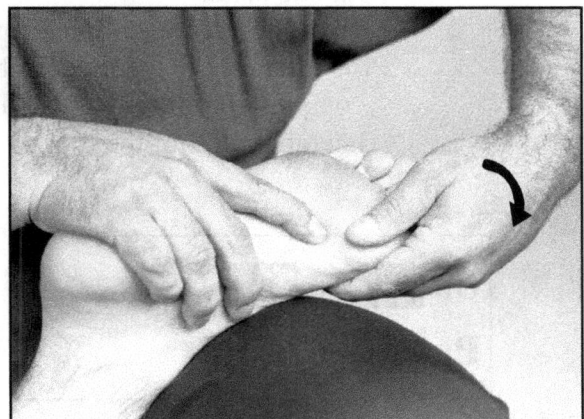

Flexed Second-Fourth Metatarsals (M2-4)

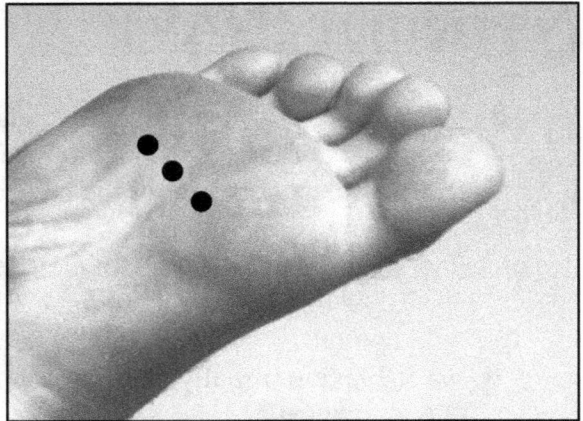

Tender Pts.   On the plantar proximal heads of the metatarsals 2-4 at base/head of MT joints.

Treatment   Patient prone with foot elevated. Operator is beside patient stabilizing foot with one hand while flexing and supinating the shaft of the metatarsal that is being treated. About 3 kg force is applied.
Flexion- moderate of the metatarsal on the tarsal
Supination- moderate of the shaft of the metatarsal

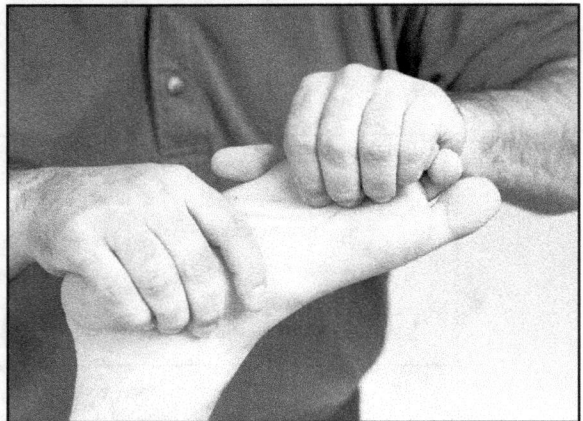

| F | |
| Su | |

Flexion Fifth Metatarsal (M5)

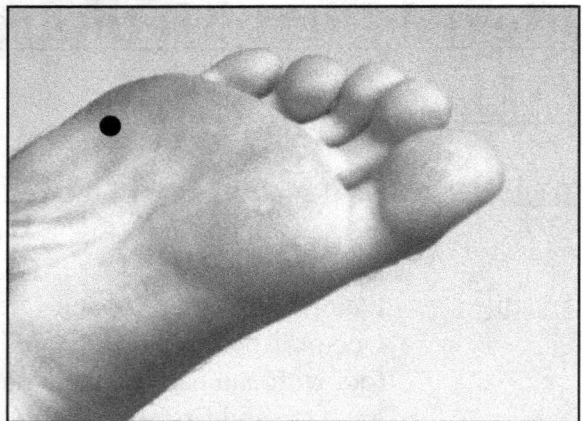

Tender Pt.   On the medial shaft of the fifth metatarsal, proximal to the MP joint.

Treatment   Patient prone with foot elevated. Operator is beside patient, squeezing the foot from medially and laterally with one hand.
Supination- of the fifth metatarsal
Pronation- of big toe induced by compression from the medial and lateral aspects of the foot

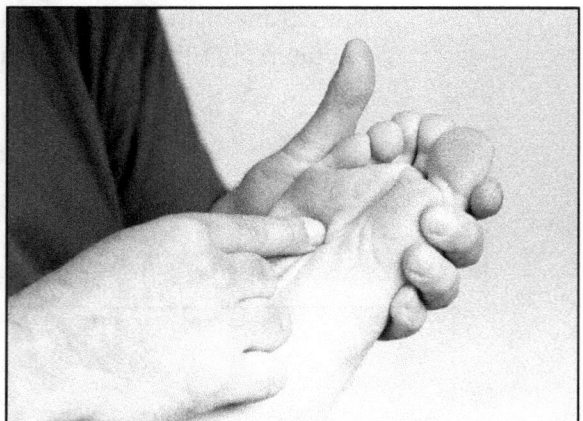

| Su | |
| Pr | |

Bunion or Lateral Sesamoid (LSE)

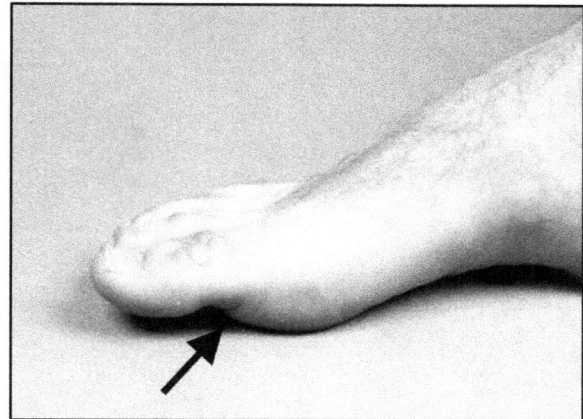

Tender Pt.   On the medial first MT joint. It can be on the dorsal or plantar surface of the foot.

Treatment   Flexion- dorsi or plantar flex towards tender point

Rotation- internally or externally for comfort

Abduction- great toe away from mid-line of body

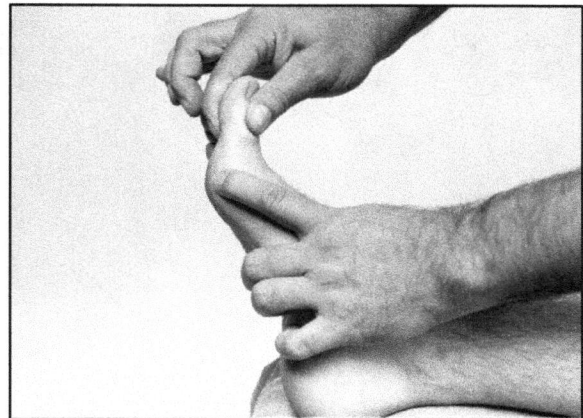

F/E	
Ri/Re	
Ab	

Notes

Cranial Tender Points

In general, treatment of tender points of the cranium follow the principle of approximation of structures towards the tender point. The pressure required is usually mild to moderate. The most important elements of treatment are exact localization of the tender point and correct introduction of force direction and amplitude.

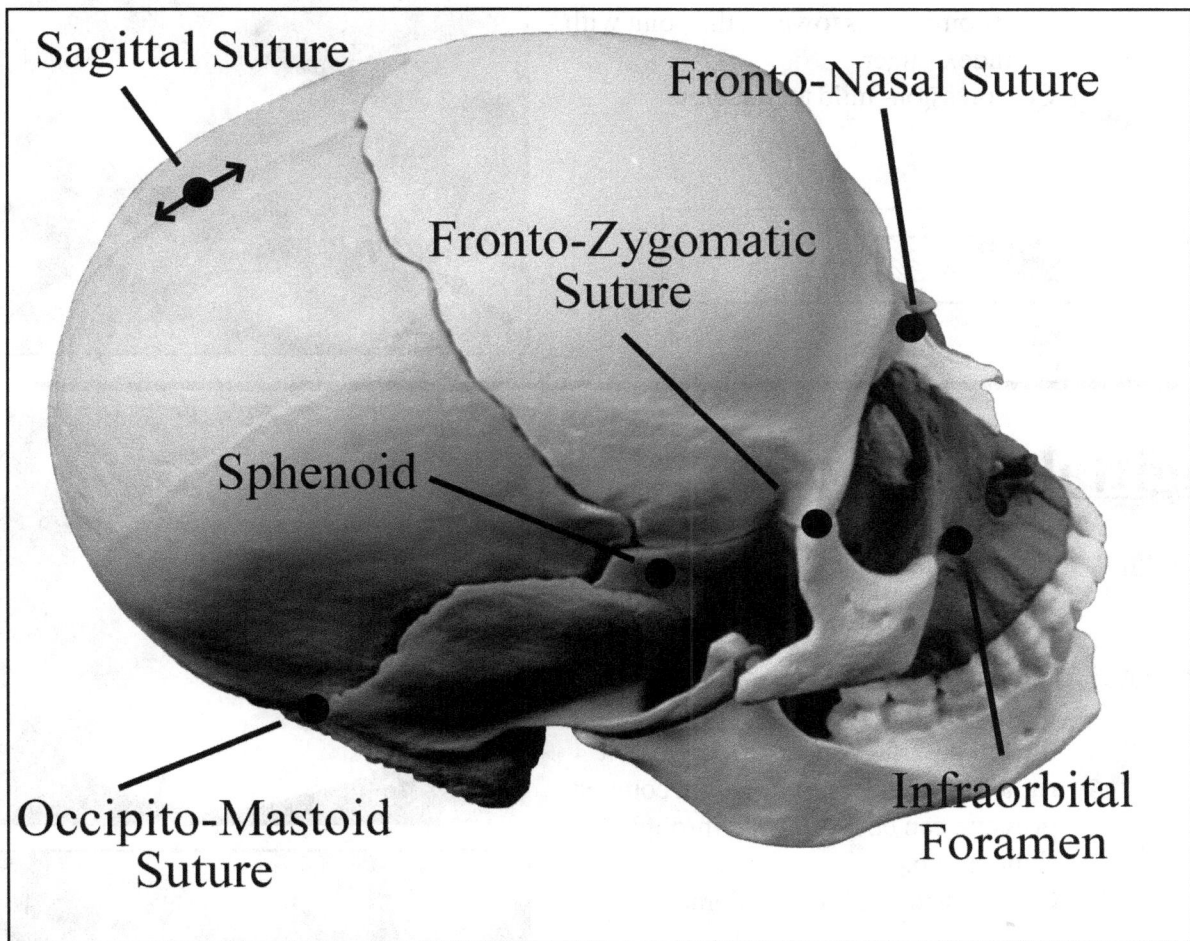

Sagittal Suture

Fronto-Nasal Suture

Fronto-Zygomatic Suture

Sphenoid

Occipito-Mastoid Suture

Infraorbital Foramen

Occipito-Mastoid Suture (OMS)

Tender Pt.   Along suture at the junction of the occipital and mastoid bones. The tender point is best palpated with the index finger

Treatment   Apply pressure from forearm on frontal bone down toward the tender point (compression). Pressure from the other hand compresses towards the point with the index finger
Compression- mild to moderate

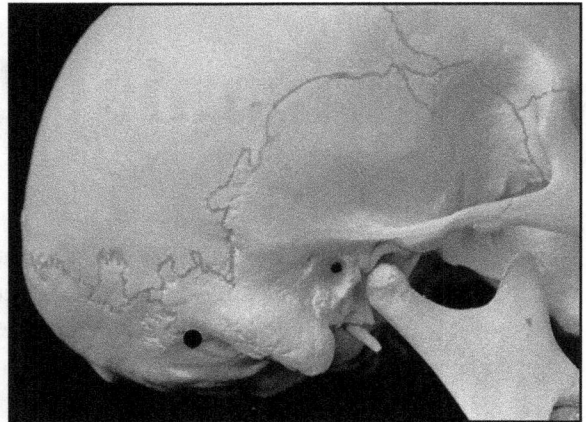

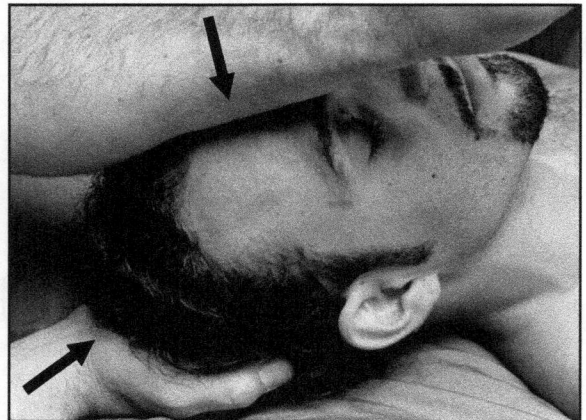

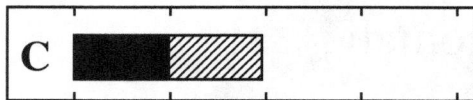

Sagittal Suture (SS)

Tender Pt.   Located on the parietal bone along either side of the sagittal suture.

Treatment   Patient supine. The operator's thumb pushes from left to right approximating the left parietal bone in direction of a right sided tender point. Slight counter-pressure can be introduced through the right thumb.
Compression- mild to moderate

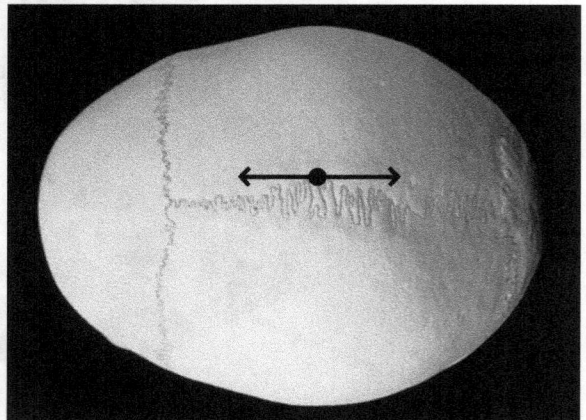

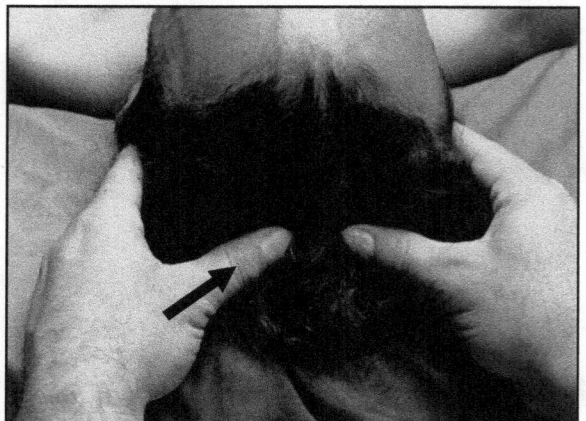

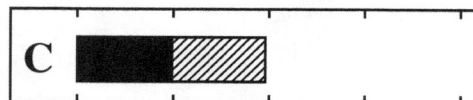

Infraorbital Foramen (IOF)

Tender Pt.   In area of infra-orbital foramen, approximately halfway between zygomatico-maxillary suture and nasal cavity

Treatment   Patient supine. Carefully place thenar/hypothenar eminences over the frontal and zygomatic bones while fingers interdigitate. Apply pressure by squeezing thenar/hypothenar eminences together towards midline while tractioning in an anterior direction, attempting to "lift the bones." ("Tenting")
Compression- mild to moderate
Traction- mild anterior

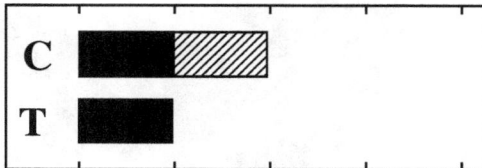

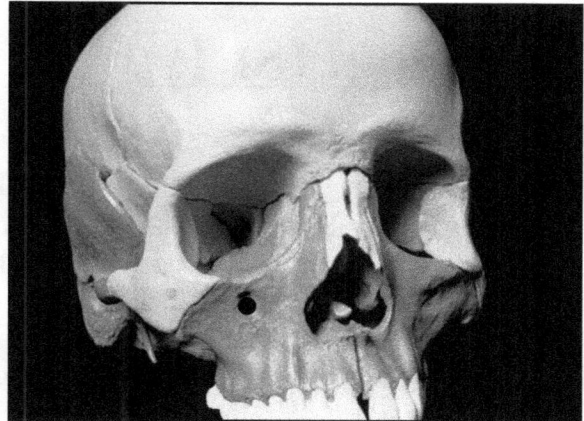

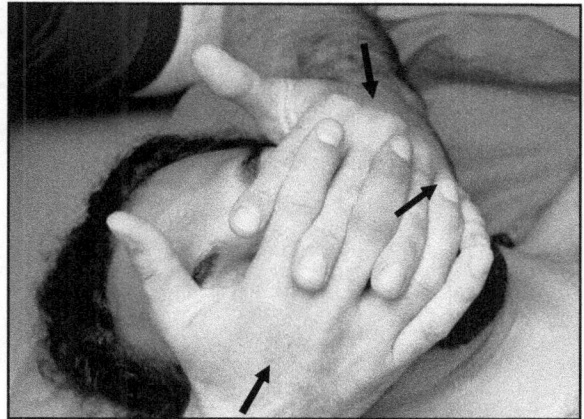

Fronto-Nasal Suture (FNS)

Tender Pt.   At the fronto-nasal suture. Usually midline but may be located to either side of center.

Treatment   Patient supine. Apply pressure with thumb towards tender point (from left to right for a right tender point). The left forearm may assist gently in providing pressure medially. The right index finger is used for "fine-tuning" rather than pure pressure.
Compression- mild

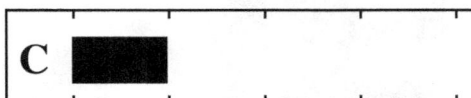

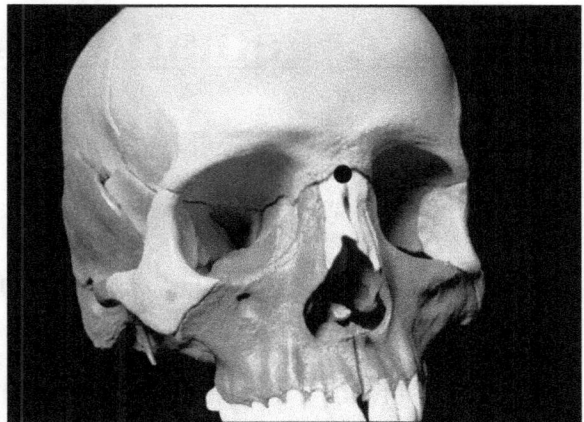

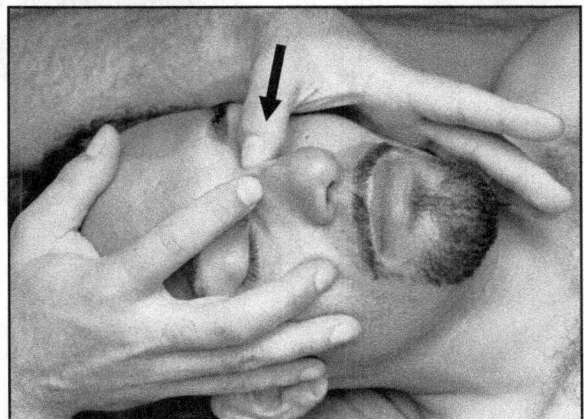

Sphenoid (SPH)

Tender Pt.   Over greater wing of sphenoid

Treatment   Patient supine. The broadly placed hand pushes on the opposite side of the sphenoid in the direction of the tender point while the fingers placed over the tender point assist in stabilization. Pressure is induced through the opposite hand (pisiform bone) at the greater wing of the sphenoid in the direction of the tender point.
Compression- mild

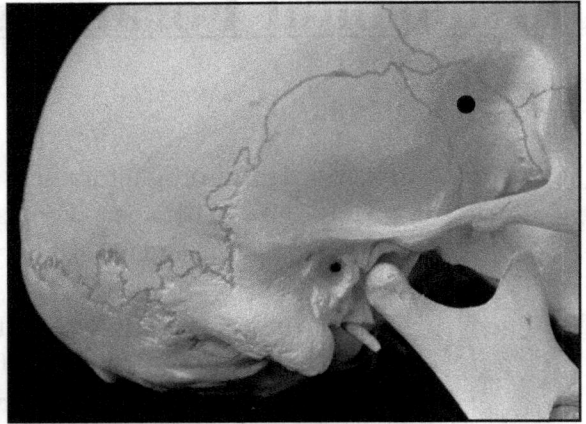

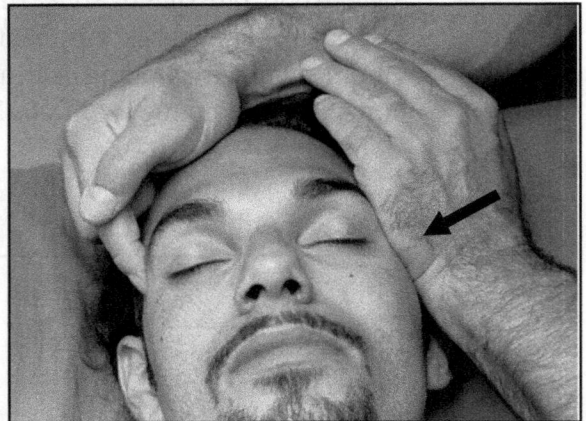

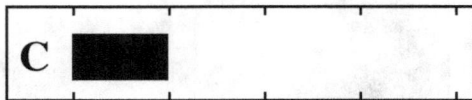

C	████			

Fronto-Zygomatic Suture (FZS)

Tender Pt.   Overlying the fronto-zygomatic suture.

Treatment   Patient supine. The superior hand cradles the frontal bone as broadly as possible. The inferior thenar eminence is placed broadly over the zygoma. Both hands are approximated towards the point with slight anterior/posterior translation or shearing force.
Compression- mild to moderate

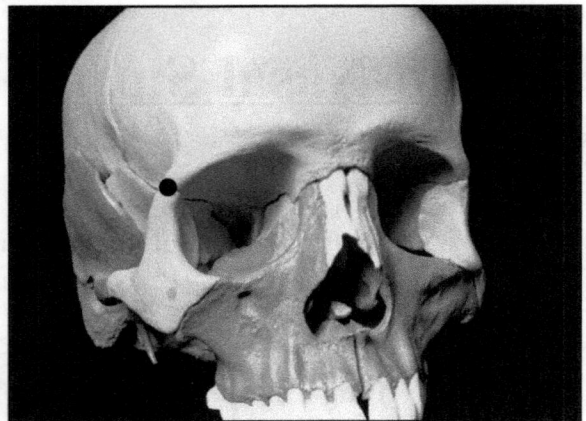

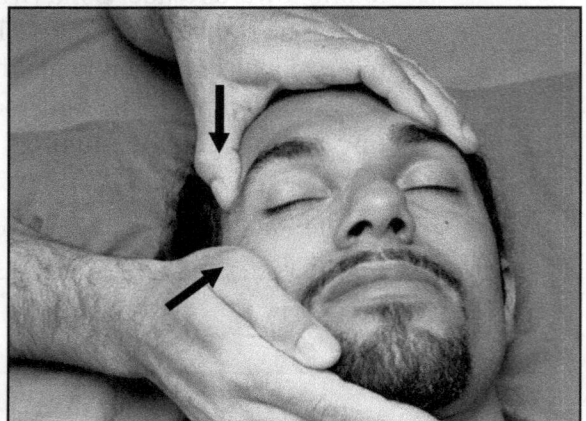

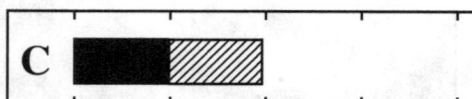

C	████	▨▨▨		

OSTEOPATHIC CLINICAL PROBLEM SOLVING

The osteopathic approach to patient care considers the patient as an integrated whole with dynamic interplay between structure and function. Problem solving begins with a detailed history and physical examination to consider all the possible etiologies related to the patient's present health status. From an osteopathic perspective, old illnesses and injuries leave their imprint on body structure and function, often making the patient more vulnerable to developing future problems. Even routine childbirth is considered to be a potential 'traumatic' event in the patient's history.

In the osteopathic approach to problem solving, patient complaints are evaluated independently, problem by problem, as well as in light of their relation to the patient's overall structure and function. This requires focused local inspection as well as examination of more distal structures for relevant clinical associations. Distal structures may have associations which can be primary (causal) or contributory to the area of the patient's chief complaint. Such associations can be mechanically linked (e.g. tendonitis), neurologically linked (e.g. radiculopathy), or viscerally linked (e.g. angina).

For example, a shoulder problem may be due to local injury to the capsule or to myotendinous insertions, or to more distal problems in the rib cage, thoracic outlet, cervical spine, gall-bladder, or opposite hip extensors. A good history and physical examination should serve to screen out these and other potential problems and help localize the clinical nature of the patient's chief complaint.

Management of problems associated with the patient's chief complaint may require emergent intervention or specialty referral for appropriate medical treatment as with an acute cholelithiasis or a stress fracture. In these situations, osteopathic manipulative treatment may also be helpful as adjunctive care. In many cases, osteopathic diagnosis and treatment alone will be effective in addressing the various mechanical, neurologic and visceral aspects and interelationships associated with the patient's chief complaint.

OSTEOPATHIC PROBLEM SOLVING MATRIX

An osteopathic screening examination with the goal of determining where the patient's problem areas are, should include: 1) gait analysis and 2) regional tests to evaluate structural landmarks, tissue resistance, and mobility. In addition to standard neurologic and orthopedic assessments, specific osteopathic tests should be carried out to evaluate possible nerve entrapment and myofascial/dural tension signs. Various approaches to locating areas of primary restrictions in the body and visceral structures can also be incorporated including palpating peripheral reflections of the cranial rhythmic impulse (CRI) or 'listening' techniques. Additionally, viscerosomatic or Chapman's reflexes may be present, also signifying the presence of visceral influences within the patient's musculoskeletal system.

Osteopathic scanning and segmental examinations further localize problems to specific areas and define their structural and functional characteristics so that specific therapeutic measures can be applied. Management of the whole patient requires consideration of the inter-relationships of the various problems identified, as well as further work-up of any potential health risks.

EXAMINATION OF THE ADULT PATIENT

SCREENING TESTS: To locate problems, regionally

1. Gait Analysis:

Forefoot pronation
Ankle eversion
Knee rotation and extension
Hip extension
Pelvic weight shift/mobility

Lumbar side bending
Thoracic cage mobility
Shoulder position
Arm swing
Head position

2. Static Landmarks

Scoliosis
Kyphosis
Lordosis

Head
Shoulder
Scapula
Iliac crest
Trochanter
Feet

3. Tissue Resistance to Pressure

4. Dynamic Testing

Standing
Pelvis
    Stork Test
Lumbar
    Rotation
    Side bending
    Flexion
Lower extremity
    Hip shift
    One leg stand
    Knee extension
Sitting
Upper extremity
    Forearm
    Pronation
Thoracic cage
    Side bending
    Rotation
    Flexion/extension
Cervical spine
    Side bending
    Rotation
    Flexion/extension

Supine
Pelvis
    Traction test
    Pelvic rock
Thoracolumbar spine
    Sit-up test
Head and cervical spine
    Head lift
    Jaw abduction
    Vault hold
Upper extremity
    Shoulder abduction
Lower Extremity
    Side bending
Costal cage
    Respiratory motion
    Sternal compliance
Prone
Pelvis
    Sacral rock
    Hip extension
Thoracic spine
    Push-up
Side-lying
Lower extremity
    Hip abduction

SCANNING TESTS: To localize segmentally, exact areas of dysfunction

1. Global "Listening"

2. Following Reflections of Peripheral CRI to Most Proximal Area of Assymetric Function

3. Tissue Texture Abnormalities

Moisture
Hardness

Temperature
Color

SEGMENTAL TESTING: To characterize dysfunction structurally and functionally

Ankle/foot
Knee
Hip/groin
Pelvis
Sacrum

Lumbar spine
Thoracic spine
Rib cage
Cervical spine
Head

Sternoclavicular
Acromioclavicular
Glenohumeral
Elbow
Wrist/hand

Course Schedule
Counterstrain A- Day 1

8:00 am   (*9:00 am*)   Course information and introductions

8:15 am   (*9:15 am*)   Definitions
- Counterstrain
- Tender points versus trigger points
- Indirect Technique

8:30 am   (*9:30 am*)   History of counterstrain technique

8:45 am   (*9:45 am*)   Counterstrain theory: Models and mechanisms

9:15 am   (*10:15 am*)   Counterstrain treatment method

9:45 am   (*10:45 am*)   Break

10:00 am   (*11:00 am*)   *Table Session-* Anterior thoracic tender points, diagnosis and treatment

11:45 am   (*12:45 pm*)   Lunch

1:00 pm   (*2:00 pm*)   *Table Session-* Posterior thoracic tender points, diagnosis and treatment

2:45 pm   (*3:45 pm*)   Break

3:00 pm   (*4:00 pm*)   *Table Session-* Anterior rib cage tender points, diagnosis and treatment

5:00 pm   (*6:00 pm*)   Adjourn

Course Schedule
Counterstrain A- Day 2

8:00	am	(*9:00 am*)	Questions
8:15	am	(*9:15 am*)	*Table Session*- Posterior rib cage tender points, diagnosis and treatment
9:45	am	(*10:45 am*)	Break
10:00	am	(*11:00 am*)	*Table Session*- Anterior cervical tender points, diagnosis and treatment
11:45	am	(*12:45 pm*)	Lunch
1:00	pm	(*2:00 pm*)	*Table Session*- Posterior cervical tender points, diagnosis and treatment
2:30	pm	(*3:30 pm*)	Break
3:00	pm	(*4:00 pm*)	*Table Session*- Anterior lumbar and pelvic tender points, diagnosis and treatment
5:00	pm	(*6:00 pm*)	Adjourn

Course Schedule
Counterstrain A- Day 3

8:00 am (*9:00 am*) Questions

8:15 am (*9:15 am*) *Table Session-* Posterior lumbar tender points, diagnosis and treatment

9:45 am (*10:45 am*) Break

10:00 am (*11:00 am*) *Table Session-* Posterior pelvic tender points, diagnosis and treatment

11:45 am (*12:45 pm*) Lunch

1:00 pm (*2:00 pm*) Clinical integration and problem solving

3:00 pm (*4:00 pm*) Adjourn

Course Schedule
Counterstrain B- Day 1

8:00 am   (*9:00 am*)   Course information and introductions

8:15 am   (*9:15 am*)   Review counterstrain theory and method

9:45 am   (*10:45 am*)   Break

10:00 am   (*11:00 am*)   *Table Session-* Axillary region tender points, diagnosis and treatment

11:45 am   (*12:45 pm*)   Lunch

1:00 pm   (*2:00 pm*)   *Table Session-* Shoulder region tender points, diagnosis and treatment

2:45 pm   (*3:45 pm*)   Break

3:00 pm   (*4:00 pm*)   *Table Session-* Upper extremity tender points, diagnosis and treatment

5:00 pm   (*6:00 pm*)   Adjourn

Course Schedule
Counterstrain B- Day 2

8:00　am　　(*9:00 am*)　　　　Questions

8:15　am　　(*9:15 am*)　　　　*Table Session*- Wrist and hand tender points, diagnosis and treatment

9:45　am　　(*10:45 am*)　　　Break

10:00　am　　(*11:00 am*)　　*Table Session*- Hip tender points, diagnosis and treatment

11:45　am　　(*12:45 pm*)　　Lunch

1:00　pm　　(*2:00 pm*)　　　*Table Session*- Anterior knee tender points, diagnosis and treatment

2:45　pm　　(*3:45 pm*)　　　Break

3:00　pm　　(*4:00 pm*)　　　*Table Session*- Posterior knee tender points, diagnosis and treatment

4:00　pm　　(*5:00 pm*)　　　*Table Session*- Ankle and foot tender points, diagnosis and treatment

5:00　pm　　(*6:00 pm*)　　　Adjourn

Course Schedule
Counterstrain B- Day 3

8:00   am   *(9:00 am)*   Questions

8:15   am   *(9:15 am)*   *Table Session-* Ankle and foot tender points, diagnosis and treatment
                                                (continued)

9:45   am   *(10:45 am)*   Break

10:00 am   *(11:00 am)*   *Table Session-* Cranial tender points, diagnosis and treatment

11:45 am   *(12:45 pm)*   Lunch

1:00   pm   *(2:00 pm)*   Clinical integration and problem solving

3:00   pm   *(4:00 pm)*   Adjourn

SFIMMS SERIES IN NEUROMUSCULOSKELETAL MEDICINE

AUTHORS: Harry Friedman D.O., Wolfgang Gilliar D.O., Jerel Glassman D.O.

Osteopathic approaches to patient care offer the practitioner a variety of problem-solving and treatment options. Palpatory skill development establishes a basis for diagnostic assessment of neuromusculoskeletal function and its integrative role in maintaining health and overcoming disease. Osteopathic treatment and problem-solving skills apply a holistic approach that considers the therapeutic response of the whole patient. A variety of diagnostic and treatment methods have been developed to maximize outcomes.

This series of Osteopathic manipulative medicine texts presents a comprehensive course of instruction, including theory, palpation, diagnosis, and treatment. The thoughtful student will appreciate the detail and clarity of topic presentation and the sequence of skills development. Quality close-up photographic visuals accurately depict the table sessions using human and anatomic models.

COUNTERSTRAIN APPROACHES IN OSTEOPATHIC MANIPULATIVE MEDICINE

* Basic and intermediate level instructional manual
* Theoretical principles of indirect technique and spontaneous release by positioning
* Diagnostic application of tender point palpation for each body region
* Multiple therapeutic procedures presented for each tender point

MYOFASCIAL AND FASCIAL-LIGAMENTOUS APPROACHES IN OSTEOPATHIC MANIPULATIVE MEDICINE

* Basic and advanced level instructional manual
* Detailed connective tissue anatomy and physiology
* Theoretical principles of myofascial and fascial-ligamentous release
* Diagnostic and treatment approaches for each body region, including a myofascial screening exam
* Release enhancing maneuvers and multiple operator techniques
* Includes approaches of Dr.'s Ward, Chila, Becker, Barral and Sutherland

OSTEOPATHIC MANIPULATIVE MEDICINE APPROACHES TO THE PRIMARY RESPIRATORY MECHANISM

* Basic, intermediate, and advanced level instructional manual
* Anatomic relations and physiologic principles underlying the cranial concept
* Palpation exercises designed to facilitate diagnostic touch throughout the body
* Diagnostic and treatment approaches focus on fluid, membranous (dural), muscular, articular and bony aspects of the cranial mechanism, including a cranial screening exam
* Includes multiple operator techniques and approaches to infants and children

FUNCTIONAL METHODS IN OSTEOPATHIC MANIPULATIVE MEDICINE

* Presents Functional Methods approach developed by William L Johnston DO FAAO
* 2 basic level courses to cover all body regions
* Presents a unique palpation based understanding of the functional relationships between all body regions
* Diagnostic principles based on passive motion testing
* Treatment elegantly applies palpation based findings to restore proper relationships between body regions

email: admin@sfimms.com
www.sfimms.com

www.ingramcontent.com/pod-product-compliance
Lightning Source LLC
Chambersburg PA
CBHW072000220326
41599CB00034BA/7066